W9-AVE-046

Jane Sherwin Shapiro
1607 Brooklyn Ave.
Ann Arbor, MI 48104

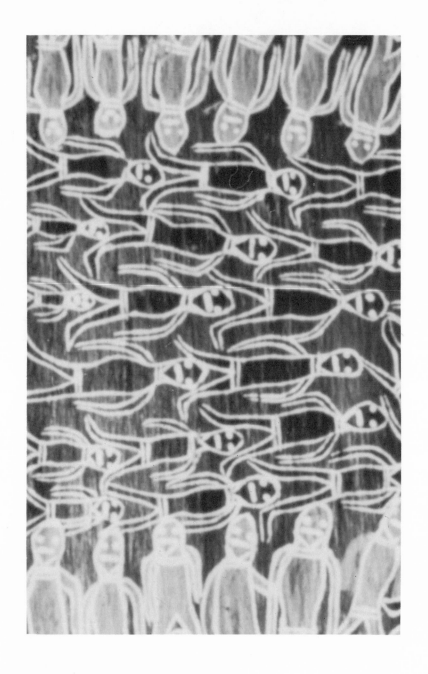

BIRTH

AN ANTHOLOGY OF ANCIENT TEXTS,

SONGS, PRAYERS, AND STORIES

EDITED BY DAVID MELTZER

North Point Press
San Francisco
1981

The author wishes to extend his gratitude to the following authors and publishers for their permission to reprint materials included in this volume. Every effort has been made to trace the ownership of copyrighted material and to make full acknowledgement of its use. If errors or omissions have occurred, they will be corrected in subsequent editions, provided that notification is submitted in writing to the publisher.
"Dinka Chant," "Song Sung by a Woman While Giving Birth," "A Mother Praises Her Baby." in *The Unwritten Song,* Volume 1, edited and with translations by Willard R. Trask. Copyright © 1966 by Willard R. Trask. Reprinted with permission of Macmillan Publishing Co., Inc. *African Myths and Tales,* by Susan Feldman. Published by Dell Publishing Co. Reprinted by permission of Presses Universitaires de France.

(continued on pages 246–248 which constitute an extension of this copyright page)

Front cover illustration is a Huichol yarn painting from Michoacan, Mexico, entitled "How the Husband Assists in the Birth of a Child." Reprinted by permission of The Fine Arts Museums of San Francisco, a gift of Mr. Peter F. Young.

Back cover illustration: Bark Painting: Djanggawul Myth, Mawalan (1908–1967), Yirrkala, Art Gallery of NSW, Sydney is printed with permission of the Art Gallery of New South Wales, Sydney, Australia and Aboriginal Artists Agency LTD, North Sydney, Australia.

Copyright © 1981 by David Meltzer
Illustrations copyright © 1981 by Jaime Robles
Printed in the United States of America
Library of Congress Catalogue Card Number: 80-82441
ISBN: Cloth, 0-86547-004-9 / Paper, 0-86547-005-7

Table of Contents

Introduction

Birth and death go together. Birth is the beginning and death is the end of life for every person. Intertwined, they are moments of intense visibility as well as profound invisibility. We regard these events with great awe. They must be attended by traditional ceremonies for the purpose of seeking happiness in this world and in the next. The baby entering life, an instant of transition from one realm to another, remains a mystery to us as it did to our ancestors. Watching a person shut his eyes to die, the animating spark suddenly gone, leaves us with another mystery, another unanswered question. Despite all that we know and have learned, we remain awe-struck before these primary moments.

The purpose of this anthology is to celebrate and gather a multi-cultural history of the awesomeness of birth, to illustrate how humankind has attempted to confront it and comprehend it. Much of the material, whether from archaic or extant cultures, approaches birth with a terror-based reverence often similar to how one faces death. But what also emerges from these texts are more subtle and essential notions of the rituals of living and dying. As we read these works we understand how important a social event birth was and how, within each social system, there were specifically designated performers assisting in the bringing forth of new life. Birth is the great multiplying force of a people's vision, their desire to duplicate their hopes into miraculous replicas. Those who participate in it are functioning in the realm of the sacred.

This book is not a manual of childbirthing nor is it a full-scale history of childbirth. There are many excellent books in those areas, a select list appears at the end of this book. This collection deals almost primarily with the impact of birth upon civilization and dwells more in the past than in the present. It is a source-book, a collection of folklore, myth, legend, song, and early anthropological studies of vanishing cultures and ways.

I've divided the book into six sections. The first is a sampler of creation myths and fabulous births. Every culture separates itself from the others through these myths which, paradoxically, bind them closer together. Metaphors of solidarity; the uniqueness of birth made into a collective legend. The second section presents a gathering of conception lore throughout the ages. Creation myths attempt to answer where the world and its special people emerge from, whereas conception lore tries to create belief structures about the origin of individual life. The third section is more expansive and deals with an enormous amount of material pertaining to amuletical magical elements people have created for protection in childbirth, to ward off death or unforeseen disasters, to shield mother and child from elaborate worlds of demons and devils. This element surrounds many births to this day. Magic is both a vulnerability and a creative gesture. Like birth and death it is an inward process which attempts to order the external borders of community reality. The fourth section presents interesting material dealing with phases of pregnancy and how many different cultures perceive it differently. The fifth, and central section, offers texts which illuminate the birth-event. In this section I've placed some works in their entirety because I felt they worked best that way and gave a full sense of a culture's concerns and approach to the birth process. It is the heart of the book and enables us all to vividly participate in some incredibly varied and well-detailed births. The sixth section presents the lore of events enacted after the birth like naming, baptizing, cauls, deaths, lullabies, and so on.

There are always important sources and acknowledgements to be made about a project like this. Most importantly, I'd like to thank Jack Shoemaker who liked this book when it was published earlier in a much different form and persisted in getting it revised and republished. I am, as usual, in enormous debt to the combined libraries of the University of California in Berkeley. Robert Hawley, of Ross Valley Books, was helpful and encouraging, as was David Guss who shared many of the enthusiasms about this anthology. And, as always, to Tina for patiently letting me grumble and pace around the house during the book's shaping and for providing warmth, insight, straightforward criticism, and advice.

Birth is the art and mystery of woman and her powerful presence is infused throughout this collection.

It is appropriate to begin with a quotation by an Abyssinian woman recorded by the anthropologist Leo Frobenius in the early twentieth century:

How can a man know what a woman's life is? A woman's life is quite different from a man's. God has ordered it so. A man is the same from the time of his circumcision to the time of his withering. He is the same before he has sought out a woman for the first time, and afterwards. But the day a woman enjoys her first love cuts her in two. She becomes another woman on that day. The man is the same after his first love as he was before. The man spends a night by a woman and goes away. His life and body are always the same. The woman conceives. As a mother she is another person than the woman without child. She carries the fruit of the night nine months long in her body. Something grows. Something grows into her life that never again departs from it. She is a mother. She is and remains a mother even though her child dies, though all her children die. For at one time she carried the child under her heart. And it does not go out of her heart ever again. Not even when it is dead. All this the man does not know; he knows nothing.

I Creation Myths and Fabulous Births

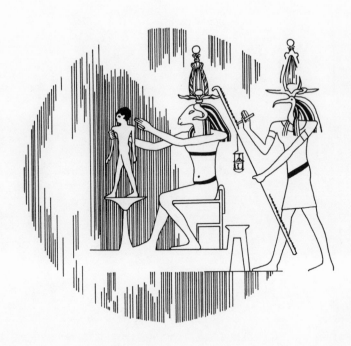

In the time when Dendid created all things,
He created the sun,
And the sun is born, and dies, and comes again;
He created the moon,
And the moon is born, and dies, and comes again;
He created the stars,
And the stars are born, and die, and come again;
He created man,
And man is born, and dies, and never comes again.

—translated by Willard Trask

1: Seruhe Ianadi

There was Kahuna, the Sky Place. The Kahuhana lived there, just like now. They're good, wise people. And they were in the beginning too. They never died. There was no sickness, no evil, no war. The whole world was Sky. No one worked. No one looked for food. Food was always there, ready.

There were no animals, no demons, no clouds, no winds. There was just light. In the highest Sky was Wanadi, just like now. He gave his light to the people, to the Kahuhana. He lit everything, down to the very bottom, down to Nono, the Earth. Because of that light, the people were always happy. They had life. They couldn't die. There was no separation between Sky and Earth. Sky had no door like it does now. There was no night, like now. Wanadi is like a sun that never sets. It was always day. The Earth was like a part of the Sky.

The Kahuhana had many houses and villages in Kahuna and they were all filled with light. No one lived on the Earth. There was no one there; nothing, just the Earth and nothing else.

Wanadi said: "I want to make people down there." He sent his messenger, a *damodede*. He was born here to make houses and good people, like in the Sky Place. That *damodede* was Wanadi's spirit. He was the Earth's first Wanadi, made by the other Wanadi who lived in Kahuna. That other Wanadi never came down to the Earth. The one that came was the other's spirit.

Later on, two more *damodede* came here. They were other forms of Wanadi's spirit.

The first Wanadi to come was called Seruhe Ianadi, the Wise. When he came, he brought knowledge, tobacco, the maraca, and the *wiriki*. He smoked and he sang and he made the old people. That was a long time before us, the people of today.

When that spirit was born, he cut his navel-cord and buried the placenta. He didn't know. Now the worms got into the placenta and they started to eat it. The placenta rotted. As it rotted, it gave birth to a man, a human creature, ugly and evil and all covered with hair like an animal. It was Kahu. He has different names. They call him Kahushawa and Odo'sha too. This man was very evil. He was jealous of Wanadi. He wanted to be master of the Earth. Because of him, we suffer now. There's hunger, sickness, and war. He's the father of all the Odoshan-komo. Now, because of him, we die.

When that old Wanadi's placenta rotted, Odo'sha sprang out of the Earth like a spear. He said: "This Earth is mine. Now there's going to be war. I'm going to chase Wanadi out of here."

He misled those peple who had just been born. He taught them to kill. There was a man fishing. He had lots of fish. Odo'sha told them: "If you kill him, you'll have lots of fish."

They killed him. Odo'sha was happy. Then the people were turned into animals as punishment.

Because of Odo'sha, Seruhe Ianadi couldn't do anything on Earth. He went back to the Sky and left the old people as animals with Odo'sha. He didn't leave any of Wanadi's people on the Earth though. That was the end of the first people.

The birth of Kahu on that old Earth is a sign to us, the people of today. When a baby is born, we should never bury the placenta. The worms get it. It rots. Another Odo'sha will come again, like in the beginning to hurt the baby, to kill it. Like what happened when Kahu fought against Wanadi for control of the Earth. When a baby is born, we put the placenta in a nest of white ants. It's safe there. The worms can't get it. Okay. Now you can bury the nest of white ants.

That was the story of the old people. That's all.

— *Marc de Civrieux*

2: The Dogon Myth of Creation

According to the Dogon the human soul is double. When a child is born the water spirit draws twin shadows on the ground. The one destined to support the feminine side of the individual is laid out first on the ground where parturition takes place. The other, which will receive the masculine side, is then sketched over the first. The newborn child is laid face down with his four limbs touching the ground and thereby takes possession of his souls. If the child is a boy the female principle will dwell on the foreskin; in case of a girl, the male principle will reside in the clitoris. These two principles are present in the individual during all of childhood. Neither wins over the other. The purpose of the rites of circumcision and excision is to force the individual to lean definitely toward the one of the two principles for which his body is the better suited. The sexual life of the individual depends on this fixation. The uncircumcised boy like the unexcised girl is both male and female. If they were to remain in the state of their first childhood, neither would feel an inclination to procreate. The boy is circumcised in order to reduce his femininity and place him definitely on the male side. A girl is excised to make her a woman. The Dogon myth of the creation of the world recounts the reason for this situation and gives the prototype of the rites of circumcision and excision.

In the beginning everything was generated by twin births: the ideal unity of being was formed by a couple. But in fact this rule has not worked ever since the first creative attempt of the God Amma. For Amma, the sole and supreme male god was forced to create a mate with whom he could unite himself to produce further offspring. Amma brought an earth woman to arise from a lump of clay. Her clitoris was made of a termite hill. When Amma tried to unite with her, the termite hill barred his way by asserting her masculinity. Amma defeated the rebellious termite hill; he cut off the obstacle and united himself with the excised earth.

This occurrence influenced the product of the union so that it was born single, in the form of a jackal. Later the god had further relations with the earth that were not disturbed and resulted in the birth of a spirit couple, *Nommo,* whose body was made of the divine seed, that is to say, water. These two creatures would little by little replace the god in insuring the progress of the universe.

It was then that the first product, the jackal, whose position was unusual because it could not procreate, committed incest with its mother, the earth, an event that was to upset the course of earthly things. The god Amma, having turned away from his wife, kneaded two clay balls out of which sprang the first human couple, who in turn procreated, giving birth to twins. But after the coming of these two beings the production of twins became a very rare exception. And it is since the birth of the first generation that the spirit couple *Nommo,* becoming the mentor of the world, minimizing the inconvenience of this new situation by creating a double soul for each being, granted through contact with the ground.

However, the first human birth brought about an event of considerable significance. The woman kneaded by Amma had intercourse with the man without having been excised. Becoming pregnant, she gave birth to twins; at that time her pains were directed to her clitoris, which fell off and went away in the shape of a scorpion, whose venom was made of both the water and the blood of parturition.

Previously her mate had been circumcised and his foreskin was transformed into *nay,* a kind of lizard.

— *Susan Feldman*

3: Eingana the Mother

(Related by Rinjeira, Djauan Tribe)

This narrative is mainly an explanation of the first appearance, and nature of, the ancestral being, Eingana. It is a Northern Territory tradition. Eingana is the great earth-mother. She is fertility itself. She is the source of all life, all forms of being.

A significant point is that, in the beginning, Eingana could not give birth in the normal manner. She had to vomit. This recalls the swallowing and vomiting acts of the Greek gods, Cronus and Zeus. Eingana both swallowed and disgorged people alive. The first nature of Eingana appears to recall some primal form of life.

Eingana, pregnant with all forms of life, and in birth travail, had to be speared, the natural opening made, to allow her to give birth. Eingana's travail to give birth here is also the explanation of the sound made by the "bull-roarer" in the Kunapipi ritual.

Eingana is the inexhaustible source of life and spirit. This explanation of her nature shows the aboriginal conception of life and spirit in continuous cycles of birth, death, and rebirth.

When this narrative was given to me, I was on the ceremonial ground of the Kunapipi ritual where initiates, under a ban of silence, and in mute subservience to the tribal elders, were awaiting their ritual birth.

That first time, the creation time, we call Bieingana. The first being we call Eingana. We call Eingana our Mother. Eingana made everything: water, rocks, trees, blackfellows: she made all the birds, flying foxes, kangaroos, and emus. Everything Eingana had inside herself in that first time.

Eingana is snake. She swallowed all the blackfellows. She took them, inside herself, down under the water. Eingana came out, she was big with everything inside her. She came out of Gaieingung, the big water hole near Bamboo Creek. Eingana was rolling about, every way, on the ground. She was groaning and calling out. She was making a big noise with all the blackfellows, everything, inside her belly.

One old-man named Barraiya has been travelling a long way. All the way he had heard Eingana crying out, rolling about and moaning. Barraiya sneaked up. He saw Eingana. He saw the big snake rolling and twisting about, moaning and calling out. Barraiya hooked up his stone-spear. He watched the big snake. He saw where he must spear her. Barraiya speared her underneath, near the anus. All blood came out of that spear wound and all the blackfellows came out after the blood.

Kandagun the dingo chased after all those blackfellows. He chased after them and split them up into different tribes and languages. When Kandagun chased the blackfellows, some flew away as birds, some bounded away as kangaroos, some raced away as emus, some became flying foxes, porcupines, snakes, everything, to get away from Kandagun.

That first time, before Barraiya speared Eingana, nothing and no one could be born as they are now. Eingana had to spew everything out of her mouth. Blackfellows had to spew everything. Children could not be born as they are now. That is why Barraiya had to spear Eingana.

The old-man Barraiya had been travelling from the east across to the west. After he speared Eingana, the old-man went back to his place Barraiyawim. There he painted himself on a rock. He turned into the blue-winged kookaburra.

Eingana made the big Boolmoon River, she made the Flying Fox River and the Roper River. Every river she made. We have water now. That's why we are alive.

Eingana made Bolong the Rainbow-Snake. In the first time when Eingana swallowed blackfellows, she spewed them out and these black-fellows became birds, they became Bonorong the brolga, Janaran the jabiroo, Baruk the diver. Eingana spewed out blackfellows who became Koopoo the kangaroo, Kandagun the dingo, Galwan the goanna, Nabi-ninbulgai the flying fox. All these birds, animals, all these things, Eingana took back. She talked: "I think that all you fellows have to follow me, you have to go my way." Eingana took them all back. She swallowed them again. She let them go in the water as snakes, as Bolong the Rainbow-Snake.

No one can see Eingana. She stays in the middle water. She has a hole there. In the rain-time, when the floodwater comes, Eingana stands up out of the middle of the floodwater. Eingana looks out at the country. She lets go all the birds, snakes, animals, children belonging to us; Eingana lets all these things go out of her.

Eingana floats along on the floodwater. She stands up and looks out at the country. She lets every kind of life, belonging to her, go. When the floodwater goes down Eingana goes back to her camp again. She comes back no more. No matter cold weather or hot weather, she does not come out. Next rain-time she comes out and lets go everything that belongs to her: snakes, birds, dingoes, kangaroos, blackfellows, everything.

Eingana keeps hold of a string, a sinew called Toon. This string is joined to the big sinew of any kind of life, behind the heel. Eingana keeps hold of that string all the time. Because we call her mother, you see. When we die Eingana lets that string go. I die. I die forever. My spirit, Malikngor, follows the way of Bolong.

It might be that I die in another place. That one, Malikngor, my spirit goes back to my country, where I was born. Everyone's spirit does this.

Eingana gives back spirit to man and woman all the time. She gives them this spirit in children. Eingana gives spirit a little bit first time to lubra, then more and more. You cannot find this spirit yourself. That one Eingana, or Bolong, has to help you.

If Eingana died, everything would die. There would be no more kangaroos, birds, blackfellows, anything. There would be no more water, everything would die.

— Roland Robinson

4: The Birth of Moses

Old as Jochebed was, she regained her youth. Her skin became soft, the wrinkles in her face disappeared, the warm tints of maiden beauty returned, and in a short time she became pregnant.

Amram was very uneasy about his wife's being with child; he knew not what to do. He turned to God in prayer, and entreated Him to have compassion upon those who had in no wise transgressed the laws of His worship, and afford them deliverance from the misery they endured, while He rendered abortive the hope of their enemies, who yearned for the destruction of their nation. God had mercy on him, and He stood by him in his sleep, and exhorted him not to despair of His future favors. He said further, that He did not forget their piety, and He would always reward them for it, as He had granted His favor in other days unto their forefathers. "Know therefore," the Lord continued to speak, "that I shall provide for you all together what is for your good, and for thee in particular that which shall make thee celebrated; for the child out of dread whose nativity the Egyptians have doomed the Israelite children to destruction, shall be this child of thine, and he shall remain concealed from those who watch to destroy him, and when he has been bred up, in a miraculous way, he shall deliver the Hebrew nation from the distress they are under by reason of the Egyptians. His memory shall be celebrated while the world lasts, and not only among the Hebrews, but among strangers also. And all this shall be the effect of My favor toward thee and thy posterity. Also his brother shall be such that he shall obtain My priesthood for himself, and for his posterity after him, unto the end of the world."

After he had been informed of these things by the vision, Amram awoke, and told all unto his wife Jochebed.

His daughter Miriam likewise had a prophetic dream, and she related it unto her parents, saying: "In this night I saw a man clothed in fine linen. 'Tell thy father and thy mother', he said, 'that he who shall be born unto them, shall be cast into the waters, and through him the waters shall become dry, and wonders and miracles shall be performed through him, and he shall save My people Israel, and be their leader forever'."

During her pregnancy, Jochebed observed that the child in her womb was destined for great things. All the time she suffered no pain, and also she suffered none in giving birth to her son, for pious women are not included in the curse pronounced upon Eve, decreeing sorrow in conception and in childbearing.

At the moment of the child's appearance, the whole house was filled with radiance equal to the splendor of the sun and the moon. A still greater miracle followed. The infant was not yet a day old when he began to walk and speak with his parents, and as though he were an adult, he refused to drink milk from his mother's breast.

Jochebed gave birth to the child six months after conception.

—Louis Ginzberg

5: The Mystery of Sperm

From the occult standpoint, then, the spermatozoon is the carrier of the archetype. It is a little *ark* in which the seeds of life are carried upon the surface of the waters that at the appointed time they may replenish the earth. A triad of forces — spiritual, psychical, and material — are contained within the head of the sperm. This triad originated from the three great centers of man referred to exoterically as the heart, the head, and the navel. The sperm also contains the Logoi, or generating gods — the Builders — those who are to establish their foundations in the deep and upbuild their thrones in the midst of the waters. With them come also the hierarchies of celestial powers — the star spirits — pioneer gods going forth to build new worlds. In the ovum is the plastic stuff which is to be molded by the heavenly powers. In the ovum lies the sleeping world, awaiting the dawn of manvantaric day. In it lurk the Chhaya forms of time and place. Suddenly above the dark horizon of the ovum appears the blazing spermatic sun. Its ray shoots into the deep. The mother ocean thrills. The sperm follows the ray and vanishes into the mother. The germ achieves immortality by ceasing of itself and continuing in its progeny. The mother ovum is fertile. She produces the lesser sun — the Demiurge, or the Builder. The law is established. The Builder calls forth the world form. The One becomes two; unity is swallowed up in diversity. Fission begins; by cleavage the One releases the many. The gods are released. They group around the Poles. The zones are established. Each of the gods releases from himself a host of lesser spirits. The germ layers come into being. The gods gather about the North Pole. The shape is bent inward upon itself. The mineral becomes a plant, the plant an animal, and the animal a man. The Builders take up their places in the organs and the parts, and the Father Cell beholds the work from His hidden place, and He sees that it is good.

—*Manly Palmer Hall*

6: The Birth of the Bodhisattva

There lived once upon a time a king of the Shakyas, a scion of the solar race, whose name was Shuddhodana. He was pure in conduct, and beloved of the Shakyas like the autumn moon. He had a wife, splendid, beautiful, and steadfast, who was called the Great Maya, from her resemblance to Maya the Goddess. These two tasted of love's delights, and one day she conceived the fruit of her womb, but without any defilement, in the same way in which knowledge joined to trance bears fruit. Just before her conception she had a dream. A white king elephant seemed to enter her body, but without causing her any pain. So Maya, queen of that godlike king, bore in her womb the glory of his dynasty. But she remained free from the fatigues, depressions, and fancies which usually accompany pregnancies. Pure herself, she longed to withdraw into the pure forest, in the loneliness of which she could practice trance. She set her heart on going to Lumbini, a delightful grove, with trees of every kind, like the grove of Citraratha in Indra's Paradise. She asked the king to accompany her, and so they left the city, and went to that glorious grove.

When the queen noticed that the time of her delivery was approaching, she went to a couch overspread with an awning, thousands of waiting-women looking on with joy in their hearts. The propitious constellation of Pushya shone brightly when a son was born to the queen, for the weal of the world. He came out of his mother's side, without causing her pain or injury. His birth was as miraculous as that of Aurva, Prithu, Mandhatri, and Kakshivat, heroes of old who were born respectively from the thigh, from the hand, the head, or the armpit. So he issued from the womb as befits a Buddha. He did not enter the world in the usual manner, and he appeared like one descended from the sky. And since he had for many aeons been engaged in the practice of meditation, he now was born in full awareness, and not thoughtless and bewildered as other people are. When born, he was so lustrous and steadfast that it appeared as if the young sun had come down to earth. And yet, when people gazed at his dazzling brilliance, he held their eyes like the moon. His limbs shone with the radiant hue of precious gold, and lit up the space all around. Instantly he walked seven steps, firmly and with long strides. In that he was like the constellation of the Seven Seers. With the bearing of a lion he surveyed the four quarters, and spoke these words full of meaning for the future: "For enlightenment I was born, for the good of all that lives. This is the last time that I have been born into this world of becoming."

—*Ashvaghosha*

7: Creation of Man by the Mother Goddess

(. . .) her breast,
(. . .) the beard,
(. . .) the cheek of the man.
(. . .) and the raising
(. . .) of both eyes, the wife and her husband.
(Fourteen mother-) wombs were assembled

(Before) Nintu.
(At the ti)me of the new moon
(To the House) of Fates they called the votaries.
(. . .) Ea came and
(Kneel)ed down, opening the womb.
(. . .) . . . and happy was his countenance.
(. . . bent) the knees (. . .),
(. . .) made an opening.
She brought forth her issue
Praying.
Fashion a clay brick into a core,
Make . . . stone in the midst of (. . .);
Let the vexed rejoice in the house of the one in travail!
As the Bearing One gives birth,
May the mo(ther of the ch)ild bring forth by herself!

—*translated by E. A. Speiser*

8: The Birth of Tarzan

A few days later, as Clayton was working in the afternoon on an addition to the cabin, he saw monkeys racing through the trees in terror. The cause of their alarm came swiftly and boldly through the jungle as if it had decided to quit spying on them and to attack. It walked semierectly, occasionally placing the backs of its fists on the ground. It was a huge anthropoid ape intent on its goal: the killing of the human male. It growled deeply but gave a low bark now and then, its four great yellow brown sharp-pointed canines gleaming wetly. It was huge, standing when erect about six feet three inches high and weighing about 350 pounds. Long black hair covered it except on its face and chest, which were black-skinned. Its forehead was low and slanting, and its black eyes were set under a bulge of bone. The jaws jutted forward, and the lips were thin and black.

(Burroughs gives the above description of the *mangani*. Clayton merely wrote that it rushed at them.)

Clayton, having grown careless lately, had left his firearms in the cabin.

Alice had been sitting by the door while she knitted another dress for the baby to come. He shouted at her to run inside, and she started to obey him, then looked back. The brute was between the cabin and her husband, who was starting to swing at it with his ax.

He shouted at her to lock the door, but she ran on inside and grabbed the only rifle in the cabin, a Lee-Matson. She ran out just in time to see the ax ripped out of her husband's grip and sent spinning toward the bush. Then the great ape was dragging her husband toward his huge canine teeth.

Alice pointed the rifle and pulled the trigger. The recoil knocked her down, but she was up at once and then frantically trying to work the bolt and eject the cartridge. John had tried to get her to learn how to operate a rifle, but she had always been afraid of firearms and had refused to learn. And now the nightmare creature had dropped her husband and was advancing on her. It stood upright on its two legs, its arms held out toward her.

She screamed and at the same time struggled with the mechanism of the rifle. Then it was on her and she had fallen beneath its crushing bulk.

John Clayton leaped up from the ground and ran to the bodies. The ape lay on top of the woman; both were motionless; a bloody hole in its back showed where Alice's bullet had gone. John rolled the heavy corpse off and cried out when he saw the blood all over her dress. But an examination showed him that the blood was the ape's.

Gently he carried her into the cabin and there tried to bring her back to consciousness. Despite his efforts, she did not wake for an hour. Yet she had not a mark on her except for the bruise given by the rifle's recoil.

When she opened her eyes, her first words revealed that her mind was affected. She thought she was in their London town house on Carlton House Terrace. She was sure that she had just had a particularly frightening dream during which she had been attacked by horrible beasts.

That night, while a leopard screamed near their door, a son was born.

Clayton did not record the exact minute of birth. He did indicate it as Thursday, November 22, 1888, shortly after midnight of November 21. The future "Lord Greystoke" was ushered into the world under the zodiacal sign of Sagittarius, the Archer. But his birth date was so close to the sign of Scorpio that he was on the "cusp," the line (as imaginary as the equator) where one sign ends and the next sign begins. If we did not have Clayton's record, we would still be able to deduce the infant's birth as being on or near November 22. He shared so many of the basic characteristics of Scorpio, the passionate, and Sagittarius, the hunter.

Sagittarius, the centaur with the bow, could not be a better symbol of the half-animal, half-man who was to be so deadly an archer and killer. He also had a lively, if sometimes cruel, sense of humor (Mark Twain was a Sagittarian). This was to be evidenced by his trickster pranks among animals and men alike. He was also frank, impulsive, restless, had much intellectual curiosity, and loved the outdoors and animals. Sagittarius is the sign associated with long journeys, and Tarzan was to out-Ulysses Ulysses in his wanderings. (Also, Thursday's child has far to go.) This sign is intimately coupled with the tendons of the muscular system, very appropriately for the strongest man in the world. Sagittarians usually have much better than average health, and their recuperative powers are amazing. Sagittarians, somehow, are always at the right place at the

21

right time, and the penchant of coincidence to occur in Tarzan's neighborhood has been noted by many.

A Scorpio is no halfway person; he has extreme likes and dislikes. He is liable to want the world to agree with him, rather than to adapt to the world. He is a fierce competitor. He attracts persons and *situations* (thus Tarzan has a double magnetism for coincidence exceeding the probabilities of chance). He can be aroused to great anger but also to intense sensitivity and kindness.

Scorpio rules the sexual-reproductive organs. Scorpio men exude sexual power, and the readers of the biography by Burroughs have noted the many attempts of women to seduce Tarzan. A Scorpio is also ingenious, creative, a true friend, and a dangerous enemy. He is very deep and mysterious, no matter how unreserved he seems to be.

The young Greystoke was to be all of the above.

Clayton performed the delivery, his only assistance the medical books he had brought along and his determination that the baby would live. He had laudanum and morphine to lessen her pain, but he was afraid to give her much because of weakening her pelvic and stomach muscles and also affecting the baby. Fortunately, the infant came swiftly. Alice did not begin screaming until fifteen minutes before the baby was out, and after that he dosed her with laudanum. He cut the umbilical cord and did all that was necessary and some things that were not. In 1888, the use of soap and water and carbolic acid during birth was well known, though not always practiced. The discoveries of the Frenchman Pasteur, the Englishman Lord Lister, and the Hungarian Semmelweis had reduced fatalities during childbirth, and Lord Greystoke used their knowledge that night in the little cabin on the coast of West Africa. It was a grim, painful, anguished, bloody, and lonely night, but it was successful—as far as the baby was concerned.

Alice never recovered from the double shock of the attack and the birth. Though she was physically healthy, she usually lived in a dream England. Clayton did not attempt to break her delusion. She was happy and could not have been a better mother.

—*Philip José Farmer*

9: The Birth of Apollonius of Tyana

Now he is said to have been born in a meadow, hard by which there has been now erected a sumptuous temple to him; and let us not pass by the manner of his birth. For just as the hour of his birth was approaching, his mother was warned in a dream to walk out into the meadow and pluck the flowers; and in due course she came there and her maids attended to the flowers, scattering themselves over the meadow, while she fell asleep lying on the grass. Thereupon the swans who fed in the meadow set up a dance around her as she slept, and lifting their wings, as they are wont to do, cried out aloud all at once, for there was somewhat of a breeze blowing in the meadow. She then leaped up at the sound of their song and bore her child, for any sudden fright is apt to bring on a premature delivery. But the people of the country say that just at the moment of the birth, a thunderbolt seemed about to fall to earth and then rose up into the air and disappeared aloft; and the gods thereby indicated, I think, the great distinction to which the sage was to attain, and hinted in advance how he should transcend all things upon the earth and approach the gods, and signified all the things that he would achieve.

—Philostratus

10: Flowers of the Christ-Child

Many flowers are believed to have first sprung into being or to have first burst into blossom at the moment when Christ was born, or very near that auspicious hour.

The Sicilian children, so Folkard tells us, put pennyroyal in their cots on Christmas Eve, "under the belief that at the exact hour and minute when the infant Jesus was born this plant puts forth its blossom." Another belief is that the blossoming occurs again on Midsummer Night.

In the East the Rose of Jericho is looked upon with favor by women with child, for "there is a cherished legend that it first blossomed at our Saviour's birth, closed at the Crucifixion, and opened again at Easter, whence its name of Resurrection Flower."

Gerarde, the old herbalist, tells us that the black hellebore is called "Christ's Herb," or "Christmas Herb," because it "flowereth about the birth of our Lord Jesus Christ."

Certain varieties of the hawthorn also were thought to blossom on Christmas Day. The celebrated Abbey of Glastonbury in England possessed such a thorn tree, said to have sprung from the staff of Joseph of Arimathea, when he stuck it into the ground, in that part of England, which he is represented as having converted. The "Glastonbury Thorn" was long believed to be a convincing witness to the truth of the Gospel by blossoming without fail every Christmas Day.

—*Alexander Francis Chamberlin*

11: Ovid's Account of Princess Myrrha

Ovid recounts in his *Metamorphoses* (10.298–518) the legend of how the princess Myrrha, daughter of King Kinyras of Cyprus, conceived an incestuous love for her father, which with the aid of her nurse she contrived to satisfy. First on a festival night when her father was drunk with wine, and then eleven nights following, repeatedly, until the king, desiring at last to know what his mistress looked like, brought in a light and (as Ovid tells) "beheld his crime and his daughter."

Appalled and speechless, Kinyras reached for his sword; but his daughter had already fled. She had conceived, and full of shame prayed the gods to let her be nowhere, among neither living men nor the dead. And some divinity—Zeus possibly, more probably Aphrodite—in pity turned her into the tree that weeps the fragrant gum known as myrrh.

In due time the growing child inside caused the tree to swell in mid-trunk, where it cracked and gave forth its burden—whom naiads gently received, laid on a bed of leaves, and anointed with his mother's tears.

12: *From the conception the increase...*

From the conception the increase,
From the increase the thought,
From the thought the remembrance,
From the remembrance the consciousness,
From the consciousness the desire.

The word became fruitful;
It dwelt with the feeble glimmering;
It brought forth night:
The great night, the long night,
The lowest night, the loftiest night,
The thick night, to be felt,
The night to be touched,
The night not to be seen,
The night ending in death.

From the nothing the begetting,
From the nothing the increase,
From the nothing the abundance,
The power of increasing,
The living breath.
It dwelt with the empty space and produced the atmosphere which is
    above us.

II Conception Lore

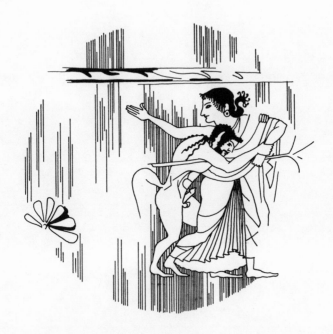

The Law (of the universe) is as here explained; but men are always incapable of understanding it, both before they hear it, and when they have heard it for the first time. For though all things come into being in accordance with this Law, men seem as if they had never met with it, when they meet with words (theories) and actions (processes) such as I expound, separating each thing according to its nature and explaining how it is made. As for the rest of mankind, they are unaware of what they are doing after they wake, just as they forget what they did while asleep.

—Heracleitus of Ephesus

13: Predicting the Sex of Unborn Baby

Far back in history another idea developed which was to play a large part in later theories of sexuality. In the sixth century B.C. the Greek philosopher Parmenides said that male babies are formed in the right side of the mother's body and females in the left. This idea was to impress Hippocrates, as perhaps was also the belief of Empedocles (fifth century B.C.) that males, being warmer, are produced in the warmer part of the uterus. The "Father of Medicine" (about 400 B.C.) described both tests and physical signs whereby fetal sex could be determined. He believed that boys develop on the right side of the uterus (i.e. on the warmer side of the body), and girls on the left. Therefore, he said, if the fetus were a boy, the right eye of the mother would be brighter and clearer and her right breast would be larger and of a particular shape. In addition, her complexion would usually be clear. If the unborn baby were of the opposite sex, the mother's left eye would be larger and brighter, the left breast larger, and she would probably have a freckled face.

Pliny the Elder contended that a woman pregnant with a boy had a better color. If her baby was to be a girl, however, the woman moved with difficulty and her legs were swollen. Soranus, who lived in the second century, quoted (with some amplification) Hippocrates' physical signs, as well as others, but scorned them as unreliable and untrue in what is perhaps the earliest recorded skepticism regarding the prognosis of fetal sex. Galen (A.D. 131–201), however, whether or not aware of Soranus' rejection of the Hippocratic theory, seems to have fully accepted it. Pulverized birthwort and honey were mixed and applied on a pessary of wool. If the woman's saliva became sweet, she could expect a son; if bitter, a daughter. Obviously this method, like many others, not only had no basis in fact but was highly subjective and hence was doubly fallacious. Paulini simply examined the saliva: if it was yellow or red and viscous, it indicated a male; if white and watery, a female (1714). A modern saliva test, although much more refined, appears also not always to be reliable (Ellin and MacDonald, 1956).

Galen suggested that parsley be placed on the woman's head without her knowledge; if thereafter she first spoke to a male, it meant that she would have a son. Priscian (fourth century) and Constantine the African (eleventh century) approved of this method, but Joubert listed the test among the *erreurs populaires*.

Peter Bayer suggested that a grain of salt be bound on the woman's breast over night; "if the salt remains dry, she has conceived a male; if it is moist and liquefied, a female" (Bayrus, 1561). A modern German peasant might lay salt on the head of a sleeping woman; the first name she speaks after awakening will reveal the sex of her child (Bachtold-Stäubli, 1930).

It is a curious fact that none of the medical writers mentioned dreams as indicators of fetal sex. On the other hand, of course, dreams often had great significance for the credulous layman. In Russia, when a pregnant woman dreamed of a fountain or spring she expected a girl; of a knife or hatchet, a boy. A dream that the stone fell from a ring forecast the birth of a son but also his death. Dreams of the death of a pregnant woman, or of a knife or ax, were in Europe another indication that the unborn child was a male, while in India the same meaning was attached to dreams of lotus blossoms and mango trees.

To Maori natives, the dreams of the father are significant; human heads or skulls decorated with *kotuku* plumes mean a boy, while *huisa* feathers signify a girl. In Southeast Asia, when the pregnant woman has dreamed of a number, she and her female friends sit up for as many successive nights as the number indicates, awaiting the cry of a bird or beast. If the cry is heard by all present, it indicates, dependent on the direction from which it comes, whether the child will be a boy (from the right) or a girl (from the left). Should the sound be heard from in front or behind, disaster threatens the baby. In this case the husband is quickly summoned to drive away the animal or bird. If thereafter the sound comes from the left or right, the child is safe.

In Albania the croaking of a raven or the nocturnal crowing of a rooster presaged the birth of a boy, while the cry of an owl told an Albanian or French mother that she would have a daughter. As Hovorka and Kronfeld suggest, girls could scarcely have been welcome; the owl's call was also an omen of impending death. On the other hand, in Dalmatia the owl's screech foretold a boy. African sorcerers informed the credulous that if a rooster looked at the door when he crowed, he was predicting the birth of a daughter. If he turned his back on the door, a son might be expected. Armenian women tore a hole in a cobweb. If the spider mended the hole quickly, a son was on the way, while a leisurely repair job meant a girl. And in medieval Italy the answer was sought from a lizard whose tail had been cut off. If the tail did not regenerate, there would be an abortion. If one new tail grew from the old stump, the woman would have a boy. A double new tail (which may occur) meant a girl.

Medieval England had a charming test. The expectant mother was simply offered a lily and a rose. Selection of the lily foretold that her unborn child was a boy; the rose indicated a girl. If, as seems likely, she knew the significance of the flowers, then no one could blame her for so pleasantly expressing her preference for a son or daughter.

—Thomas Rogers Forbes

14: The Angel and the Unborn's Soul

The soul and body of man are united in this way: When a woman has conceived, the Angel of the Night, Lailah, carries the sperm before God, and God decrees what manner of human being shall become of it—whether it shall be male or female, strong or weak, rich or poor, beautiful or ugly, long or short, fat or thin, and what all its other qualities shall be. Piety and wickedness alone are left to the determination of man himself. Then God makes a sign to the angel appointed over the souls, saying, "Bring Me the soul so-and-so, which is hidden in Paradise, whose name is so-and-so, and whose form is so-and-so." The angel brings the designated soul, and she bows down when she appears in the presence of God, and prostrates herself before Him. At that moment, God issues the command, "Enter this sperm." The soul opens her mouth, and pleads: "O Lord of the world! I am well pleased with the world in which I have been living since the day on which Thou didst call me into being. Why dost Thou now desire to have me enter this impure sperm, I who am holy and pure, and a part of Thy glory?" God consoles her: "The world which I shall cause thee to enter is better than the world in which thou hast lived hitherto, and when I created thee, it was only for this purpose." The soul is then forced to enter the sperm against her will, and the angel carries her back to the womb of the mother. Two angels are detailed to watch that she shall not leave it, nor drop out of it, and a light is set above her, whereby the soul can see from one end of the world to the other. In the morning an angel carries her to Paradise, and shows her the righteous, who sit there in their glory, with crowns upon their heads. The angel then says to the soul, "Dost thou know who these are?" She replies in the negative, and the angel goes on: "These whom thou beholdest here were formed, like unto thee, in the womb of their mother. When they came into the world, they observed God's Torah and His commandments. Therefore they became the partakers of this bliss which thou seest them enjoy. Know, also thou wilt one day depart from the world below, and if thou wilt observe God's Torah, then wilt thou be found worthy of sitting with these pious ones. But if not, thou wilt be doomed to the other place."

In the evening, the angel takes the soul to hell, and there points out the sinners whom the Angels of Destruction are smiting with fiery scourges, the sinners all the while crying out "Woe! Woe!" but no mercy is shown unto them. The angel then questions the soul as before, "Dost thou know who these are?" and as before the reply is negative. The angel continues: "These who are consumed with fire were created like unto thee. When they were put into the world, they did not observe God's Torah and His commandments. Therefore have they come to this disgrace which thou seest them suffer. Know, thy destiny is also to depart from the world. Be just, therefore, and not wicked, that thou mayest gain the future world."

Between morning and evening the angel carries the soul around, and shows her where she will live and where she will die, and the place where she will be buried, and he takes her through the whole world, and points out the just and the sinners and all things. In the evening, he replaces her in the womb of the mother, and there she remains for nine months.

When the time arrives for her to emerge from the womb into the open world, the same angel addresses the soul, "The time has come for thee to go abroad into the open world." The soul demurs, "Why dost thou want to make me go forth into the open world?" The angel replies: "Know that as thou wert formed against thy will thou shalt die, and against thy will thou shalt give account of thyself before the King of kings, the Holy One, blessed be He." But the soul is reluctant to leave her place. Then the angel fillips the babe on the nose, extinguishes the light at its head, and brings him forth into the world against his will. Immediately the child forgets all his soul has seen and learnt, and he comes into the world crying, for he loses a place of shelter and security and rest.

—*Louis Ginzberg*

Ancient Egyptian

15: The Hymn of Aton

Creator of seed in women,
Thou who makest fluid into man,
Who maintainest the son in the womb of his mother,
Who soothest him with that which stills his weeping,
Thou nurse (even) in the womb,
Who givest breath to sustain all that he has made!
When he descends from the womb to breathe
On the day when he is born,
Thou openest his mouth completely,
Thou suppliest his necessities.
When the chick in the egg speaks within the shell,
Thou givest him breath within to maintain him.
When thou has made him his fulfillment with the egg to break it,
He comes forth from the egg to speak at his completed (time);
He walks upon his legs when he comes forth from it.
                            — *translated by John A. Wilson*

16: Positions and Reasons

The Position of the Private Parts

At the beginning of the world it had been the Creator's intention to place both men's and women's genitals on their foreheads so that they might be able to procreate children easily. But the otter made a mistake in conveying the message to that effect; and that is how the genitals come to be in the inconvenient place they are now in.

The Reason for There Being No Fixed Time
for Human Beings to Copulate

Anciently the Creator summoned all the birds and beasts, the gods and devils together, in order to instruct them on the subject of copulation. So the birds and all the others of every sort assembled, and learnt from the Creator when to copulate, and when to give birth to their young.

Then the Creator said to the horse: "Oh! thou divine ancestor of horses! It will be well for thee to copulate one spring, and to give birth to thy young in the spring of the following year; and thou mayest eat any of the grass that may grow in any land!" At these words, the horse was delighted, and forthwith trotted out. But, as he rose, he kicked God in the forehead. So God was very angry, and pressed his hand to his head, so much did it hurt him.

Meanwhile, the ancestor of men came in, and asked saying: "How about me? When shall I copulate?" To which God, being still angry, replied: "Whenever you like!" For this reason, that race of creatures which is called man copulate at all times. (Translated literally. Told by Ishanashte, 12th July, 1886.)

— Basil H. Chamberlain

17: From *The Tibetan Book of the Dead*

There are four kinds of birth: birth by egg, birth by womb, supernormal birth, and birth by heat and moisture. Amongst these four, birth by egg and birth by womb agree in character.

As above said, the visions of males and females in union will appear. If, at that time, one entereth into the womb through the feelings of attachment and repulsion, one may be born either as a horse, a fowl, a dog, or a human being.

If [about] to be born as a male, the feeling of itself being a male dawneth upon the Knower, and a feeling of intense hatred towards the father and of jealousy and attraction towards the mother is begotten. If [about] to be born as a female, the feeling of itself being a female dawneth upon the Knower, and a feeling of intense hatred towards the mother and of intense attraction and fondness towards the father is begotten. Through this secondary cause — [when] entering upon the path of ether, just at the moment when the sperm and the ovum are about to unite — the Knower experienceth the bliss of the simultaneously-born state, during which state it fainteth away into unconsciousness. [Afterwards] it findeth itself encased in oval form, in the embryonic state, and upon emerging from the womb and opening its eyes it may find itself transformed into a young dog. Formerly it had been a human being, but now if it have become a dog it findeth itself undergoing sufferings in a dog's kennel; or [perhaps] as a young pig in a pigsty, or as an ant in an ant-hill, or as an insect, or a grub in a hole, or as a calf, or a kid, or a lamb, from which shape there is no [immediate] returning. Dumbness, stupidity, and miserable intellectual obscurity are suffered, and a variety of sufferings experienced. In like manner, one may wander into hell, or into the world of unhappy ghosts, or throughout the Six *Lokas,* and endure inconceivable miseries.

Those who are voraciously inclined towards this (i.e. *sangsaric* existence), or those who do not at heart fear it, — O dreadful! O dreadful! Alas! — and those who have not received a *guru's* teachings, will fall down into the precipitous depths of the *Sangsara* in this manner, and suffer interminably and unbearably. Rather than meet with a like fate, listen thou unto my words and bear these teachings of mine at heart.

Reject the feelings of attraction or repulsion, and remember one method of closing the womb-door which I am going to show to thee. Close the womb-door and remember the opposition. This is the time when earnestness and pure love are necessary. As hath been said, "Abandon jealousy, and meditate upon the *Guru* Father-Mother."

As above explained, if to be born as a male, attraction towards the mother and repulsion towards the father, and if to be born as a female, attraction towards the father and repulsion towards the mother, together with a feeling of jealousy [for the one or the other] which ariseth, will dawn upon thee.

For that time there is a profound teaching. O nobly-born, when the attraction and repulsion arise, meditate as follows:

"Alas! what a being of evil *karma* am I! That I have wandered in the *Sangsara* hitherto, hath been owing to attraction and repulsion. If I still go on feeling attraction and repulsion, then I shall wander in endless *Sangsara* and suffer in the Ocean of Misery for a long, long time, by sinking therein. Now I must not act through attraction and repulsion. Alas, for me! Henceforth I will never act through attraction and repulsion."

Meditating thus, resolve firmly that thou wilt hold on to that [resolution]. It hath been said, in the *Tantras*, "The door of the womb will be closed up by that alone."

O nobly-born, be not distracted. Hold thy mind one-pointedly upon that resolution.

18: Zuñi Shrines

Previous to the birth of a child, if a daughter is desired, the husband and wife, sometimes accompanied by a doctress or a female relative, visit the Mother rock,[1] on the west side of To'wa yäl'länně (Corn Mountain). The pregnant woman scrapes a small quantity of the rock into a tiny vase made for the purpose and deposits it in one of the cavities in the rock, and they all pray that the daughter may grow to be good and beautiful and possess all virtues, and that she may weave beautifully and be skilled in the art of making pottery. If a son is desired, the couple visit a shrine higher up the side of the mountain, in a fissure in the same rock, and sprinkle meal and deposit *te'likinawe,* with prayers that a son may be born to them and that he may be distinguished in war and after death become great among ancestral gods. Should the prayers offered at the shrines be not answered, it is believed that the heart of one or the other of the couple is not good. There is also another shrine most sacred to the Zuñis to which parents desiring sons resort. This shrine is on the summit of a low mound in a narrow valley and consists of a stone slab about one foot square, slightly raised from the ground by loose stones. Three stones, two round and one several inches long, symbolizing the male generative organs, are placed upon the slab, the long one pointing to the east.

Another resort for women in this condition is a queer-looking enclosure by the side of the trail leading to the peach orchards of To'wa yäl'länně. It is formed by a stone wall some 2½ feet high at the west end, the space within being 2½ by 6 feet. Two of the largest stones of the wall project into the interior. The wall slopes unevenly on each side and is only a foot high at the east end. When a daughter is desired, one or the

1. The base of this rock is covered with symbols of the *a'sha* (vulva) and is perforated with small excavations. The Zuñis are not an exception among aboriginal peoples in respect to phallic worship.

other of the couple or both visit this place and the woman, passing into the enclosure, breaks off a bit from each of the projecting rocks. These bits are afterward powdered and put into water and drunk by the woman. It is believed that a daughter is sure to be the result if the heart is good.

—Matilda C. Stevenson

19: The Stork and Babies

Dutch, German, and Scandinavian mothers especially tell their children that babies are brought by the stork. They say, too, that the stork, when depositing the baby, bit the mother's leg, causing her to stay in bed for some time.

In its very name the stork carries a tradition of love. The English word comes from the Greek *storgé*, meaning "strong natural affection," and in the sacred language of Hebrew the stork appears literally as "the pious one."

Several factors combined in creating the belief in the stork as the bringer of babies. First, there was the bird's remarkable tenderness towards its young and old. Legends grew up which described how the young ones looked after the aged, blind, and weak parents; how they carried them around on their own wings and fed them.

People watched the stork's care in making its home and noted how it loved to return to the same spot each year. Soon, the stork's very presence was considered a sign of good fortune. Indeed, German peasants often encouraged it to build its nest on the roof of their house, putting a wagon wheel there for a foundation. The stork soon used it for that very purpose.

The bird's regular trip abroad added to the mystery. At the time, people knew nothing of the migratory habit of birds, and legend assumed that during the winter storks went to Egypt and there changed into men. It was believed that the stork once had been a human being.

Finally, there was the fact that storks loved water and frequented swamps, marshes, and ponds. Ancient tradition held that it was in those watery places that the souls of unborn children dwelt.

It was easy to link all these beliefs and superstitions, to make the stork, so conspicuous in appearance, all-important in the propagation of man.

—*R. Brasch*

20: Words Spoken by Day
Enter the Bodies of Women

"Words spoken by day enter the bodies of women. Any man speaking to any woman is assisting in procreation. By speaking to a woman one fertilizes her, or at least by introducing into her a celestial germ, one makes it possible for her to be impregnated in a normal way."

(Ogotemmêli) compared a pregnant woman to an ear of millet beginning to swell within its leafy spiral. Such an ear is said to have "found its voice," perhaps by analogy with a fertilized woman, who also has found a voice, that is, the voice of man.

But he insisted that the word, if it was to be good, must be spoken in the daytime. "Words of the day are the only good words; a word spoken by night is ill-omened." And that was why it was forbidden to talk loudly or shout or whistle in the villages by night.

"Words fly away," he said. "No one knows where they go; they are lost and that means a loss of force, for all the women are asleep at night; no ear, no sexual part will catch them."

Where could they vanish away, these words with echo and with no one to hear them? Was it right to utter, over enclosing walls, in the cracks of doors, in empty streets, words addressed to nobody?

But there was something even worse than lack of hearers. In fact in any village there are always some women who are not asleep. Words spoken by night may enter their ears. They say: "Who was that?" They never know. What is said at night is the word of an unknown speaker, falling into their wombs at random. If any woman were impregnated in this way, the embryo would be the fruit of chance, like that of promiscuous and irregular unions.

But words spoken by night do not fertilize women, and just as blows on the ground at night undo the work done by the smith on his anvil by day, so the word of the night, entering a woman's ear and passing through her throat and liver, coils itself round the womb in an inauspicious way, unwinding the efficacious spirals formed by the word of the day.

41

Bad words therefore make women temporarily unfit for procreation by destroying, or rather disturbing, the "germ of water" which is waiting to receive the contribution of the male.

But its effects were more far-reaching. Ogotemmêli had already said that the bad word did not merely occupy the womb; it passed out thence in emanations, which also played a decisive part in the act of procreation.

"Bad words smell," he said. "They affect a man's potency. They pass from the nose to the throat and liver, and from the liver to the sexual organ."

They caused a man to feel aversion.

— Marcel Griaule

III Magical Protection of Mothers and Babies from Disaster

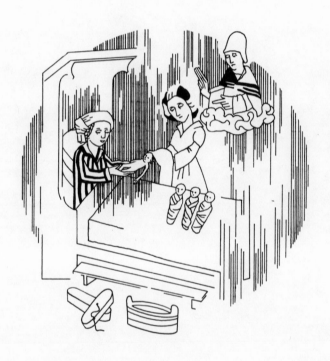

.. by the power of the holy Name
.. in the names of the angels of God
I conjure you all
kinds of Lilin, male and female,
and Demons, male and female,
by the power of the holy Name ..
      —E. A. Wallis Budge

India

21: A Song Against Miscarriage

The next song is a Satnami one and is intended to avert the danger of miscarriage. For this, a magical remedy such as the string of beads knotted ten times or indeed anything that is well tied up (it must, of course, be undone before delivery)—is bound about the waist and the people sing:

Day and night the stream flows under the moon
The true Guru has come and built his temple amid the waters
The river is very deep; no one can find the bottom of the dark pool
How has he built his temple in the middle of the stream?
Where has the boat come from, and where the paddle?
O carpenter, how did you make them in the middle of the stream?
The boat is of truth, the paddle of the word, the bamboo pole of memory
It was on the full moon day that the carpenter built the temple.

Whence is the lime and whence the cloth? How did they stick together?
The bricks are the father's, the stones are the father's; by the mother they were stuck together
It was on the full moon day that the carpenter built the temple.
Where is the lime and whence the cloth? How did they color the walls?

The lime is of silver, the cloth is of Ram, with truth they colored the walls.
In the walls they set the bones, here and there, and tied them inside
They made 3,608,000 divisions of the temple
And through it a path for the wind.

—Verrier Elwin

22: Magical Protection for a Child

Mayest thou flow away, he who comes in darkness and enters in furtively, with his nose behind him, and his face reversed, failing in that for which he came![1]

Mayest thou flow away, she who comes in the darkness and enters in furtively, with her nose behind her, and her face turned backwards, failing in that for which she came!

Hast thou come to kiss this child?
I will not let thee kiss him!
Hast thou come to silence him?
I will not let thee set silence over him!
Hast thou come to injure him?
I will not let thee injure him!
Hast thou come to take him away?
I will not let thee take him away from me!

I have made his magical protection against thee out of *clover*—that is what *sets an obstacle*—out of onions[2]—what injures thee—out of honey—sweet for men, but bitter for those who are yonder—out of the *roe* of the *abdju*-fish, out of the jawbone of the *meret*-fish, and out of the backbone of the perch.

1. Male or female ghosts, looking back as the dead look backward, and coveting a child, might slip in at night.
2. Here the magic efficacy arises out of a pun: *hedjw* "onions," and *hedjet* "what injures."

23: Gods and Goddesses of Motherhood

The number of gods and goddesses presiding over motherhood and childhood is legion; in every land divine beings hover about the infant human to protect it and assure the perpetuity of the race. In ancient Rome, besides the divinities who were connected with generation, the embryo, etc., we find, among others, the following tutelary deities of childhood:

Parca or *Partula*, the goddess of childbirth; *Diespiter*, the god who brings the infant to the light of day; *Opis*, the divinity who takes the infant from within the bosom of mother earth; *Vaticanus*, the god who opens the child's mouth in crying; *Cunina*, the protectress of the cradle and its contents; *Rumina*, the goddess of the teat or breast; *Ossipaga*, the goddess who hardens and solidifies the bones of little children; *Carna*, the goddess who strengthens the flesh of little children; *Diva potina*, the goddess of the drink of children; *Diva edusa*, the goddess of the food of children; *Cuba*, the goddess of the sleep of the child; *Levana*, the goddess who lifts the child from the earth; *Statanus*, the god, and *Dea Statina*, the goddess, of the child's standing; *Fabulinus*, the god of the child's speech; *Abeona* and *Adiona*, the protectresses of the child in its goings out and its comings in; *Deus catus pater*, the father-god who "sharpens" the wits of children; *Dea mens*, the goddess of the child's mind; *Minerva*, the goddess who is the giver of memory to the child; *Numeria*, the goddess who teaches the child to count; *Voleta*, the goddess, and *Volumnus* the god, of will or wishing; *Venilia*, the goddess of hope, of "things to come"; *Deus conus*, the god of counsel, the counsel-giver; *Peragenor* or *Agenona*, the deity of the child's action; *Camœna*, the goddess who teaches the child to sing, etc.

—*Alexander Francis Chamberlin*

24: Eilithyīa

The Greek goddess of childbirth, daughter of Zeus and Hera, according to whose will she makes childbirth easy or difficult. In Homer there is more than one goddess of the name. Just as Hera was herself often worshipped as the goddess of childbirth, so Artemis, goddess of the moon, was invoked under the title of Eilithyīa; the moon, according to ancient belief, having had great influence upon the event. The oldest seat of the worship of Eilithyīa was the island of Crete, where a grotto at Cnossus, consecrated to her, is mentioned in Homer. Next to this came the island of Delos, where she was also worshipped as a goddess of destiny. She had sanctuaries and statues in many places, being represented as veiled from head to foot, stretching out one hand to help, and in the other holding a torch as the symbol of birth into the light of the world.

—Oskar Seyffert

25: Voodoo Birth Charms

Love charms form an important category of good magic, as also charms
to aid in selling in the markets or in keeping a job or to hold the affection
of a spouse. Old men are believed to have important magical powers for
good, and one such person of great experience was pointed out who was
believed able to stop a runaway horse without putting a finger on him.
One widely spread type of charm is an *arrêt* against the *mal jok*, or evil
eye. Mention has been made of protective charms when the measures
taken to guard growing crops were discussed, and also in connection
with safeguarding the well-being of infants. The power in this latter type
of *garde* often is made to reside in a seed on a string or chain, or a cross of
beads sewed on cloth, to represent the four corners of the earth.

Because charms are the outer symbols of magic, detailed examples of
their making will give insight into the nature of charms in general. The
first of these which may be described was a *garde,* made by a *mambu,* to
relieve a pregnant woman whose milk had begun to flow before the birth
of her child—a sign that an evil spirit had been sent her by an enemy,
and that her delivery would therefore be fraught with danger. During
the séance the *mambu* was continuously possessed by her god, Ogun,
whose identity was shown by her whistling. Before the *mambu* as she
commenced her incantation were some *clairin,* lighted red candles, a
new piece of soap, incense, sulphur, garlic, light brown shoemaker's
thread, an empty bottle, a bottle filled with a green, evil-smelling lotion
called *baigne de mambu,* a chick, and three iron nails. As she tied the
cord in knots she muttered her spell; then, taking the empty bottle, she
put in it a bit of the incense, sulphur, garlic, some soap, some *clairin,*
and some *baigne de mambu.* With the knotted cord she tied a cross made
of two nails to the neck of the bottle, repeating her formula before she
put it down. Instructing the pregnant woman to take the bottle, she said:
"Speak into it and say everything you wish."

She then took the chick, opened its beak, and wrote on it with a pencil, continuing the incantation the while. With the pencil she also made marks on the thighs, the wings, the upper joints, and the leg joints before she handed it to her client with the words: "Tell it what you have to say. Tell it that you are passing on to it all your pain, everything." When she had finished, the *mambu* once again took the chick, holding its head as she described three crosses on the ground with its beak. She now put some of the earth in which she had made the crosses into a white dish, returning the chick to the woman and telling her to speak to it again, and this time to expectorate three times into its open beak as she finished. The *mambu*, holding the fowl in one hand, thereupon poured some of the mixture from the bottle, and some *clairin*, in the plate that contained the earth, lighting the *clairin* with her free hand and directing the patient to rub her nipples with it. Then she returned the bottle to the pregnant woman, telling her to recount her need to it once more, and then to cork it.

The *mambu* next chewed some of the soap and rubbed it over the cork to "seal" the bottle, saying: "When you send a letter through the mail, you seal it," and instructed the pregnant woman to place the bottle in her house and see to it that it was not uncorked, for in it was contained her life and the life of her child. "Open it before delivery and pass its contents over your abdomen." A cord was put about the waist of the woman and tied tightly, not to be untied until the growing child in her womb should cause it to break of itself. While the *garde* was being made the *mambu* sang this song:

M' pas 'ti bête,	I am not a little animal
M' pas 'ti cochon,	I am not a little pig
Pou' on cové,	That one can confine me,
Pou' on marré moin.	That one can tie me up.
Ça qui fait bien,	He who does good,
Cé bien li wé;	Good he will see;
Ça qui fait mal,	He who does evil,
Cé mal li wé.	Evil he will see.
Côté marré corde moin,	Where I tie my cord.
Yo passa la qui li.	They are stronger than it [the evil?].

The chick was released in the open countryside. Were a person to capture and eat it, the evil that had been transferred to the fowl would come to him. Many such fowl live wild in the woods, and no one touches them.

There was no hesitation in permitting spectators to witness the making of this charm; rather it was held to be good business to allow anything pertaining to a cure to become widely known. Had the transaction involved evil magic, great secrecy would have been exacted of the principals, and no others would have been present. The operation of sympathetic magic in this case—the fact that the ingredients were either cleansing or evil-smelling, for example, indicates the concept behind the charm. Similarly, the assertion that the chick which figured so prominently in the rite would carry away the *wanga* sent against the pregnant woman shows how the forces of "white" magic are manipulated to combat "black."

—Melville J. Herskovits

26: Amulet

The prayer of the Holy Sisoe for the little children who are killed by the Devil.

This is to be placed in the cradle of the child and then the Devil will not come near it.

This Saint Sisoe, with Sidor and Fidor, had waged successful wars in the country of the Arabians. He had a sister called Meletia; she had had five children, and the Devil had stolen all the five and had swallowed them; and when Meletia was to give birth to another child, Meletia, frightened of the Devil, ran away until she came to the seashore. There she found a leaden cave covered with lead and the doors of lead, wherein she placed food for a year sufficient to keep three women, as she had taken two servants with her to attend on her. When the sixth child was going to be born she was frightened of the Devil, but God, who hearkens unto all who pray unto Him with faith, when He saw how sorely grieved and frightened Meletia was on account of the Devil, listened unto her, and He sent His angel to her brother Sisoe, and he said unto him, 'Holy Sisoe, go with the fear of God against the Devil, for he has swallowed thy sister's children'. The holy Saint Sisoe went out hunting with a large number of people. When they were in the middle of the forest a terrible storm broke out and all his companions were scattered in the forest. Sisoe wandered about at the will of God until he came to the seashore to his sister Meletia. There he cried with a loud voice, 'Sister Meletia, open the door, or else I shall not be able to escape this terrible tempest'. Meletia replied, 'I will not open the door, for I am frightened of the Devil, lest he come in and steal my child, as forty days have not yet passed since its birth'. Saint Sisoe said, 'Sister Meletia, open the door, for God has sent me to hunt the Devil'. When Meletia heard these words she opened the door, and the saint entered into the cell, bringing his horse with him. The Devil, who stood by, changed himself into a millet-grain, and putting himself inside the shoe of the horse, thus entered. Thus the Devil entered the cell. Meletia kept the child in one arm and prepared food with the other. After they had eaten and gone to sleep, the Devil got up, ran to the cradle, snatched the child up, and ran away with it along the seashore through the forests. The child was screaming very loudly. When the mother heard the child screaming she got up quickly and felt with her hand in the cradle. When she found the cradle empty she cried aloud, 'Wake up, my brother, for the Devil has stolen my child'. Hearing his sister cry bitterly, the saint rose quickly, mounted his horse, took the lance in his hand, and began to pursue the Devil. On the way he came to a willow tree, and he asked, 'Hast thou, O willow of God, seen the Devil passing hereby with a child in his arms?' The willow had seen them, but it said, 'I have not seen'. Saint Sisoe then cursed the willow and said, 'O wicked willow! cursed thou shalt be, thou shalt only bloom and never bear fruit'. And he went on his way until he came to a briar, and Saint Sisoe said, 'O briar of God, hast thou seen the Devil running past with a little child in his arms?' The briar had seen them, but said, 'I have not'. Saint Sisoe cursed it, saying, 'Cursed shalt thou be, O briar! thy roots shall be where thy branches ought to be; thou shalt catch at all, and tear and be cursed by all'. And Saint Sisoe went further, following the traces of the Devil, until he came to a plane tree. 'Hast thou, O plane tree of God, seen the Devil running past with a child?' The plane tree said, 'I have not seen them, but I have heard singing on the road'. The saint replied, 'Blessed shalt thou be, and thou shalt stand in front of the church [probably to be used as the knocking-board or plank still in use in the East instead of church bells] to call the people to service and the sinners to repentance'. Then he went on further after the Devil, until he came to an olive tree standing by the seashore, and he said to it, 'Olive tree of God, hast thou seen the Devil running past with the child in his arms?' And the olive tree replied, 'Yes, I have seen him plunging into the sea, and he is playing with the fishes of the deep'. The saint replied, 'Blessed shalt thou be, from thee shall come the holy ointment, and no church shall be without thee'. The saint dismounted from his horse by the shore of the sea and knelt down and prayed to God; then he threw his hook into the sea and caught the Devil by the neck. Dragging him on to the land and beating him with a fiery sword, he said unto him, 'Give me back the children which thou hast stolen from my sister'. But the Devil replied, 'How can I return them after I have swallowed them?' And the saint replied, 'Thou must bring them up again'. The Devil said, 'Vomit thou first the milk which thou hast sucked from thy mother's breast'. And the saint prayed to God and he vomited the milk. The Devil, seeing this, got terribly frightened, and brought at once up all the six children hale and hearty, and not hurt in the least. But the saint said, 'I will not let thee free until thou swear no longer to harm man in the future'. And the Devil swore by the Lord, who created heaven and earth, that wherever he would see the name or the book of the Holy Sisoe he would have no power to harm or to hurt the people. Saint Sisoe beat him fearfully and threw him into the sea; then taking the six children he brought them to his sister, and said unto her, 'Sister! here are the children which the Devil had swallowed'. She received them with great joy, rejoicing over and over again. And this is now the prayer: 'O Evil Spirit! mayest thou be killed and cursed by the terrible and glorious name of the Trinity, and by the 360 holy fathers of the Council of Nicaea. May X. remain clear and shining through the dew of the Holy Spirit as on the day in which his mother bore him; for ever and ever, Amen'.

—Moses Gaster

27: Formulas for Childbirth

Hia' Tsunsdi'ga Dil'tadi' natanti'yi. I.
Sgĕ! Hĭsga'ya Ts'sdi'ga ha-nâ'gwa da'tûlehûⁿgû' kĭlû-gwû'. Iyû'ⁿta
agayû'ⁿlinasĭ' taya'ĭ. Eska'niyu unayĕ'histĭ' nûⁿta-yu'-tanatĭ'. Sgĕ'!
tinû'lĭtgĭ'! Tleki'yu tsûtsestâ'gĭ hwĭnagĭ'. Yû!

Sgĕ! Hige'cya ts'sdi'ga ha-nâ'gwa da'tûlehûⁿgû' kĭlû-gwû'. Iyûⁿ'ta
tsûtu'tunasĭ' tăya'ĭ. Eska'niyu unayĕ'histĭ nûⁿtayu'-tanatĭ'. Sgĕ!
tinû'lĭtgĭ'! Tleki'yu tsûtsestâ' hwĭnagĭ'. Yû!

TRANSLATION
This Is to Make Children Jump Down
Listen! You little man, get up now at once. There comes an old woman.
The horrible [old thing] is coming, only a little way off. Listen! Quick!
Get your bed and let us run away. Yû!

Listen! You little woman, get up now at once. There comes your
grandfather. The horrible old fellow is coming only a little way off.
Listen! Quick! Get your bed and let us run away. Yû!

EXPLANATION
In this formula for childbirth the idea is to frighten the child and coax it
to come, by telling it, if a boy, that an ugly old woman is coming, or if a
girl, that her grandfather is coming only a short distance away. The
reason for this lies in the fact that an old woman is the terror of all the
little boys of the neighborhood, constantly teasing and frightening them
by declaring that she means to live until they grow up and then compel
one of them to marry her, old and shriveled as she is. For the same
reason the maternal grandfather, who is always a privileged character in
the family, is especially dreaded by the little girls, and nothing will send
a group of children running into the house more quickly than the
announcement that an old "granny" of either sex is in sight.

As the sex is an uncertain quantity, the possible boy is always first addressed in the formulas, and if no result seems to follow, the doctor then concludes that the child is a girl and addresses her in similar tones. In some cases an additional formula with the beads is used to determine whether the child will be born alive or dead. In most instances the formulas were formerly repeated with the appropriate ceremonies by some old female relative of the mother, but they are now the property of the ordinary doctors, men as well as women.

This formula was obtained from the manuscript book of A'yû'ⁿinĭ, who stated that the medicine used was a warm decoction of a plant called Dalâ'nige Unaste'tsĭ ("yellow root"—not identified), which was blown successively upon the top of the mother's head, upon the breast, and upon the palm of each hand. The doctor stands behind the woman, who is propped up in a sitting position, while repeating the first paragraph and then blows. If this produces no result he then recites the paragraph addressed to the girl and again blows. A part of the liquid is also given to the woman to drink. A'yû'ⁿinĭ claimed this was always effectual.

Hia' Tsunsdi'ga Dil'tadi'natanti'yi. II.
Hitsutsa, hitsu'tsa, tleki'yu, tleki'yu, ĕ'hinugâ'ĭ, ĕ'hinugâ'ĭ! Hi'tsu'tsa, tleki'yu, gûltsû'tĭ, gûltsû'tĭ, tinagâ'na, tinagâ'na!

Higĕʻyu'tsa, higĕʻyu'tsa, tleki'yu, tleki'yu, ĕ'hinugâ'ĭ, ĕ'hinugâ'ĭ! Higĕʻyu'tsa, tleki'yu, gûⁿgu'stĭ, gûⁿgu'stĭ, tinagâ'na, tinagâ'na!

TRANSLATION
This Is to Make Children Jump Down
Little boy, little boy, hurry, hurry, come out, come out! Little boy, hurry; a bow, a bow; let's see who'll get it, let's see who'll get it!

Little girl, little girl, hurry, hurry, come out, come out! Little girl, hurry; a sifter, a sifter; let's see who'll get it, let's see who'll get it!

EXPLANATION
This formula was obtained from Takwati'hĭ, as given to him by a specialist in this line. Takwati'hĭ himself knew nothing of the treatment involved, but a decoction is probably blown upon the patient as described in the preceding formula. In many cases the medicine used is simply cold water, the idea being to cause a sudden muscular action by the chilling contact. In this formula the possible boy or girl is coaxed out by the promise of a bow or a meal sifter to the one who can get it first. Among the Cherokees it is common, in asking about the sex of a new arrival, to inquire, "Is it a bow or a sifter?" or "Is it ball sticks or bread?"

—*James R. Mooney*

28: Charm for Protection During Childbirth

(This) formidable charm dates from 1475. "For woman that travelyth of chylde, bynd thys writ to her thye." The charm itself, mostly in Latin, is an invocation. In translation it reads:

In the name of the Father † and the Son † and the Holy Spirit † Amen. † By God's grace may the Holy Cross and passion of Christ be the means of my healing. † May the five wounds of the Lord be the means of my healing. † Holy Mary bore Christ. † Holy Ann bore Mary. † Holy Elizabeth bore John. † Holy Cecilia bore Remy. † Arepo tenet opera rotas. † Christ conquers. † Christ reigns. † Christ said, Lazarus, come forth. † Christ rules. † Christ calls thee. † The world delights in thee. † The covenant longs for thee. † The Lord of vengeance is God. † Lord of battles, God, free thy servant N.[1] † The right (hand) of God established goodness. † a. g. l. a.[2] † Alpha † and Omega. † Ann bore Mary; † Elizabeth, he who went before; † Mary, Our Lord Jesus Christ, without pain and sorrow. Oh infant, whether alive or dead, come forth. † Christ calls thee to the light. † Agyos. † Agyos[3] † Christ conquers. † Christ rules. † Christ reigns. † Holy † Holy † Holy † Lord God. † Christ who art, who wert, † and who will be. † Amen. bhurnon † blictaono[4] † Christ the Nazarene. † King of the Jews, Son of God † have mercy on me. † Amen.

1. *N* for *nomen,* the name of the woman in labor.
2. AGLA is an acrostic form from the Hebrew words *attah ghibbor le'olam adhonay,* "Thou art mighty forever, O Lord." It appears often in charms.
3. Greek: "Holy, Holy."
4. I have not found a meaning for *bhurnon* and *blictaono.* Possibly they are jargon; it has also been suggested that they have Rosicrucian significance.

29: For Fertility

A pomegranate is bought in the name of Yemayá, the beautiful Yoruba moon goddess. She is the patroness of motherhood and it is usually wise to enlist her aid in matters of fertility.

The pomegranate is cut in halves, which are both covered with honey. A piece of paper with the name of the petitioner is placed between the two halves of the pomegranate, which are then put back together again. Yemayá is then invoked and asked in the same way the pomegranate is rich in health and seeds, so will the petitioner be healthy and fruitful. A blue candle is burned in Yemayá's honor every day for a month, starting with the first day of the menstruation cycle. It is not uncommon that women making this offer to this lovely goddess become pregnant during this month.

— *Migene Gonzáles-Wippler*

30: Babylonian-Assyrian Birth Omens

If a woman gives birth to two boys, famine will prevail in the land, the interior of the country will witness misfortune, and misfortune will enter the house of their father.

If a woman gives birth to two boys with one body — no union between man and wife, (that house will be reduced).

If a woman gives birth to twins united at the spine with the faces (back to back?), the gods will forsake the country, the king and his son will abandon the city.

If a woman gives birth to twins without noses and feet, the land (will be diminished).

If a woman gives birth to twins united at the sides, the land ruled by one will be controlled by two.

If a woman gives birth to twins united at the sides and the right hands are missing — attack, the enemy will destroy the produce of the land.

If a woman gives birth to three well-developed girls, the land of the ruler will be enlarged.

31: Invocation Number Fourteen for a Difficult Childbirth

There are fourteen invocations for soliciting the help of the gods in a difficult childbirth. They begin by invoking the help of Kamuy Fuchi, Fire Goddess, who dwells in the hearth of every Ainu home and inform her of the evil spirits (*wen kamuy*) impeding the childbirth. They ask her to sweep them away with the purification switches (*takusa*). If difficulties continue they seek the help of other gods; first by asking Fire Goddess to secure it and then by speaking to them directly, informing them that Fire Goddess will be coming to speak to them if she hasn't already and to please heed her supplications. Kinashut, Snake God, is called upon to coil through and clear the passage while hissing away the evil spirits. The Mortar and Elder Tree Ancestresses are also invoked. These failing, the midwife to all Ainu women, Ashke Tanne Mat, Spider Goddess, the long-fingered woman, is called upon to pull the child out. As things continue to get worse Wakka-ush Kamuy, the God of Fresh Waters, is asked to command Ami Tanne Mat, the fresh-water crab, the long-nailed woman, to put on her magic hook of iron and save the woman's life. If there is no response the long-nailed woman is summoned directly. The mother's life still in danger, the fourteenth and final invocation is made to Honpusa, Penis God, as a last resort.

Oh, Penis
Soul-Bearing God
From inside myself
  and inside the womb
there should be a baby
Gently and easily
Fire Goddess
should receive
  and hold it
    safely
Some evil spirit

working mischief in an Ainu belly
makes labor continue
   to be difficult
Urgently needed
your medicine of urine
   will clear from above
down
the belly
of the suffering Ainu
If drunk
it will clear
from above
down
any evil spirit
from the belly
and drive it forth
And then
gently and easily
Fire Goddess
shall receive it
and probably be very happy

The woman's husband now goes out to make a brew of his own urine and feces which he then gives his wife to drink. The vomiting caused by this solution serves a dual purpose. It insures a final clearing of all evil spirits from her system and also starts the exhausted pelvic muscles in motion again.

—*Marc de Civrieux*

32: The Evil Eye and Childbirth

The most probable reason for the ancient custom of veiling brides is the fear of the evil eye. The bridal veil is mentioned in the Book of Genesis (24:65) when Rebekah comes to marry Isaac, and it was a matter of course in ancient Rome that the verb meaning to veil (*nubere*) came also to mean the marrying of a woman. The same protective purpose is served by the veiling and seclusion of women in general throughout the Moslem world. Beginning perhaps with the protection of beautiful women, who naturally attract the evil eye, the implied compliment would soon be demanded by the plainer women, till all were veiled and secluded.

No sooner has a woman passed safely through the perils of her wedding than she must take thought of the dangers attendant upon pregnancy and childbirth, when the evil eye may again seek her out to cause death, abortion, birthmarks on the child, congenital defects, or the birth of monstrosities. The danger is thought to increase as pregnancy advances and becomes more apparent. This was a terror of antiquity that still shadows the peoples of modern Europe, Africa, Asia, and the Americas. The Nandis of East Africa believe that if a woman is struck by an evil eye she will abort if pregnant, and if not pregnant will develop an inflammation of the breasts.

The conception of the evil eye plays a large part in the ancient belief in maternal impressions or prenatal influences. There are many stories of women frightened by the sight of some object or animal during pregnancy, who later were delivered of a child on whose skin was marked in pigment a reproduction of the object or animal in miniature. Typical is a report written in 1686 of a pregnant woman, frightened by a mouse, whose child had the figure of a small mouse on its body. Charles Leland found that pregnant women among the Tuscan peasants of the last century were afraid of the old Roman and Etruscan relics. They feared that looking at figures which were half man and half animal, such as centaurs or the goat-legged god Pan, would cause the birth of children similarly formed. In Romania the belief is current that if a vampire sets his cold eyes on a pregnant woman, she must obtain the blessings of the Church at once or her child will grow up to be a cold-eyed vampire itself. Pregnant Chinese women must avoid looking at a hare, lest the child be born with a harelip. Wilfred T. Grenfell, who served as physician to the Labrador fishermen, encountered the same belief. To protect her unborn child from a harelip, the Labrador mother cut out and kept as an amulet a portion of the dress she was wearing when she met the hare.

There is a tale of how Hippocrates, the famous Greek physician of the fifth century B.C., saved a princess, accused of adultery because her child was black, by putting the blame on a picture of a Negro which the husband had hung on the wall of his wife's room during her pregnancy. Heliodorus of Emesa (third century after Christ) wrote a novel whose heroine was beautiful and fair-skinned. When the last chapter's happy ending revealed her as the daughter of the king and queen of Ethiopia, her unlikely complexion was attributed to a painting of the mythical Greek character Andromeda hanging in the royal bedroom, which the mother had admired during coitus. Thomas Fienus of Antwerp (1567–1631), professor of medicine at the University of Louvain, has recorded the story of a girl-child born near Pisa who was covered with hair at birth because her mother, at the time of conception, was looking at an image of St. John the Baptist which hung by the bed.

There was an English belief that the eye of the moon could cast its influence upon a pregnant woman and cause the birth of monsters. Such a monster was called a mooncalf, using the word "calf" in its meaning of a mass or protuberance, as in the calf of the leg. The deformed Caliban in Shakespeare's *The Tempest* (Act 2, Scene 2) is referred to as a "mooncalf."

In 1726 Mary Tofts, of Gadolmin in Surrey, claimed that as a result of the strange influence of a rabbit she met in the fields during pregnancy, she had begun to dream of rabbits and crave rabbit meat and had finally given birth to a litter of seventeen rabbits. The rabbits were delivered over a period of several weeks, and most of them were found, cut into pieces, in her vagina where she had placed them. Investigation by a competent obstetrician from London soon exposed the fraud. Mary confessed in prison that, after the loss of a human child by miscarriage, she had decided to win a royal pension for herself as a biological freak. Many people were quite willing to believe in the marvel, including Nathanael St. Andre, surgeon and anatomist to His Majesty George I, who lost both position and reputation in consequence. Nevertheless, the *British Medical Journal* reported a similar story in 1868. A rabbit, with eyes glaring, had jumped at a pregnant woman and frightened her badly. The child was born with an enlarged head; the mouth and face were small and rabbit-shaped, and the skin was covered with short, dark hair. The mother recovered her health, but the child died ten minutes after birth.

The *Boston Medical and Surgical Journal* in 1839 reported the case of an expectant mother, frightened by the gaze of a rattlesnake, whose child when born had an arm in shape and movements remarkably snakelike. The face and mouth resembled those of a snake, and the teeth suggested fangs. The mention of snakes filled the child, at the time of the report a man of twenty-nine, with horror and rage, especially in the "snake season." This personal reaction at least can be readily accepted. Some such report may have suggested the plot of *Elsie Venner* to the Boston physician Oliver Wendell Holmes. The heroine of this novel, published in 1861, exhibited snakelike characteristics because her mother had been bitten by a rattlesnake shortly before Elsie was born, though Holmes's purpose in writing was to show the limitations of the doctrine of free will, and not to express any great enthusiasm for the belief in prenatal influences. To complete her character Holmes endowed poor Elsie with the evil eye of the snake which had bitten her mother:

> "Elsie would have been burned for a witch in old times," said Elsie's schoolmaster to Elsie's doctor. "I have seen the girl look at Miss Darley when she had not the least idea of it, and all at once I would see her grow pale and moist, and sigh, and move round uneasily, and turn towards Elsie, and perhaps get up and go to her, or else have slight spasmodic movements that looked like hysterics — do you believe in the evil eye, Doctor?"
>
> "Mr. Langdon," the doctor said, solemnly, "there are strange things about Elsie Venner — very strange things . . . Her love is not to be desired, and" — he spoke in a lower tone — "her hate is to be dreaded."

In 1883 the *Medical Press and Circular* of London described a young man of twenty-one with congenital deformities of heart, skin, muscles, and bones, attributed to the fact that his mother had been frightened during pregnancy when a guinea pig was thrust into her face. The *International Medical Magazine* of Philadelphia reported in 1892 a child with deformed arms and legs, whose mother was frightened in pregnancy by a large turtle. According to the *Belgian Medical Press* of 1879, a pregnant woman, fascinated by the antics of a circus clown, gave birth to a child with a clown's grotesque features.

That highly respectable British medical journal *Lancet* furnished numerous cases of visual prenatal influence during the nineteenth century. In 1863 a pregnant woman who had seen the results of an amputation of the penis for cancer had a male child born without a penis. A banner year was 1890, for in that year *Lancet* reported a mother, terrified by a bull, whose child was stillborn with a cow's head; a mother, frightened by a black and white collie dog, whose child was born with a black mole studded with white hairs on the right thigh; and a mother, shocked by the sight of a crippled beggar, whose child was similarly crippled at birth.

The original Siamese twins, Eng and Chang (1811–1874), traveled about the world exhibiting themselves, and King Chowpahyi of Siam was glad to see them go, for he felt that freaks of nature brought bad luck to his country. The government of France also had forebodings and, on the grounds that the sight of the twins might cause pregnant women to produce monsters, refused an entry permit. For the same reason the exhibition of Ritta-Christina was not permitted in France. This monster, born in Sardinia in 1829, had two heads, two chests, and two pairs of arms, with a single abdomen and one pair of legs. The right torso, named Ritta, was feeble and sad, while the left, named Christina, was vigorous and gay. The parents brought Ritta-Christina to Paris, where they earned a little money by private showings, but the authorities put a stop to this in order to protect pregnant women, and the child soon died.

It will be observed that the instances of prenatal influence which occur in medical case reports are similar to the wicked, malicious use of the evil eye associated with witchcraft. No less dangerous, but less spectacular and harder to detect, are the envious glances of spinsters and childless wives who may be entirely unconscious of the harm they do. Nursing mothers must also be wary of the evil eye and not expose their breasts to view when suckling their infants, or the milk will either become scanty or make the children sick. It is true that strong emotion can affect a mother's milk, and perhaps even cause a miscarriage, but we cannot give credit to the effect of maternal impressions on the structure of the child. There is no connection between the nervous systems of mother and child, and the child is completely formed by the sixth week of pregnancy, before the pregnancy is usually recognized, and long before the period of late pregnancy when the evil eye is supposed to be most effective. Though Havelock Ellis hesitated to reject prenatal influence altogether, a noted obstetrician, Dr. Joseph B. DeLee, toward the close of a long and distinguished career, stated that he had never found any plausible connection between a nervous shock to the mother and a deformity in the child.

Marriage and pregnancy are crises in a woman's life, but if she wishes to repel the evil eye she must at all times employ prayers, amulets, and magic rites, until she has reached the age at which she no longer is able to command the admiration of the opposite sex and the envy of her own. The European women, both educated and uneducated, use methods inherited from classical antiquity, which in turn received them from a much earlier time. The women of remote and primitive tribes have their own methods. The Negro tailed headhunters of Nigeria are so called because the women wear tails made of palm fiber, tightly bound with string, which often have a wider, wheel-shaped termination. These women paint rings of white or yellow around their eyes to ward off the evil eye. The women of the Hausa tribe in northern Nigeria similarly paint red, white, or yellow rings around their eyes. A Hausa woman feels herself threatened with serious injury if her beauty is praised by any man other than her husband. To halt the effects of the evil eye she answers such dangerous compliments by saying, "I don't care, do you hear?" Doubtless this would sound rather naive to the women of America, who must keep cocktail party wolves at a polite distance with graceful phrases.

Children are especially liable to damage from the evil eye because, as Plutarch said, they have a "weak and soft temperature," or as St. Thomas Aquinas said, they have a "tender and most impressionable body," or as Roger Bacon said, they are "tender in age and complexion," or as Antonio of Cartagena said, they are of a "moist and tender constitution." With unexpected realism Antonio added that it is often difficult to determine whether young children are fascinated or are suffering from sour milk.

Accordingly, every effort must be made at the earliest possible moment to protect children from fascination. The mother, of course, has been extremely careful during her pregnancy and as soon as the child is born, takes special precautions for the infant. The ancient Romans invoked the aid of Cunina, goddess of the cradle. The ancient Persians called upon Anahita, goddess of pregnancy, birth, and lactation. Today in Persia the child's head at birth is covered with soot, preferably as soon as the head appears and before the rest of the body has been delivered. In 1809 John Cam Hobhouse, intimate friend of Lord Byron from student days at Cambridge till Byron's death in Greece, observed that in Albania a lump of mud, softened in water previously prepared with magic charms, was plastered on a newborn baby's forehead to protect it from the evil eye. More recently Albanian women have gathered after a childbirth carrying gifts of eggs, one of which was broken over the face of the baby. Defacing a child in these ways would render it less attractive, and therefore less likely to invite an envious eye.

Throughout the Balkan countries mothers wrap the heavy wooden cradles in thick woolen coverlets so that no evil eye or breath of fresh air can reach the child. Such a custom does nothing to reduce the high infant mortality, but when the children do grow sick or die it is felt that, despite every care, the evil eye has prevailed. Similarly, the peasant women of Egypt ascribe the hollow eyes, pale faces, swollen bellies, and scrawny arms and legs of their children to the evil eye rather than to malnutrition. Among the Jews of Tunis a baby was concealed from the evil eye behind thick curtains for some time after birth, and a smoking light kept burning day and night within the curtains. Indirectly, children actually do suffer from the evil eye.

The association of the evil eye with the praising of babies and young children has led to the custom of addressing them by opprobrious names, and resenting any use of flattery by admiring relatives and friends. In China children are often nicknamed *dog, hog,* or *flea* to minimize the danger of the evil eye. In India a male child may be called *dunghill, grasshopper,* or *beggar,* and a female child *blind, dusty,* or *fly.* We are following an old practice when we address our children affectionately as *scamp* or *little rascal.*

—*Edward S. Gifford*

33: Portents

An honest young woman has assured me that she has tested this receipt, which is to take three fingers of the morning urine and put it in a glass with as much red wine. Let this stand all day. If there appears at the bottom a large cloud like bean soup, it is a sign that the woman is pregnant with a boy; if it appears in the middle, it is a sign of a girl; and if there appears at the bottom only the usual urinary sediment, it is a sign that the woman is not pregnant.

—Charles Guillemeau (1620)

34: Protective Charms for Childbirth

Even in the 1840s Irish women on the delivery bed still looked for help to lines inscribed on vellum which was then tied onto the abdomen. The charm, written in the shape of a square with crosses interspersed, enumerated various holy births and closed with the SATOR formula:

```
S A T O R
A R E P O
T E N E T
O P E R A
R O T A S
```

Downright quackery was involved in the sale of a prayer to Irish immigrants as they left Queenstown. This charm was alleged to have been found in 803 in the tomb of Christ and to have been sent by the Pope to an emperor for his protection in battle.

> They who shall repeat it every day, or hear it repeated, or keep it about them, shall never die a sudden death, nor be drowned in water, nor shall poison have any effect upon them; and it being read over any woman in labor she will be delivered safely and be a glad mother.

Ulster midwives marked every outside house corner with a cross, then recited the following prayer before crossing the threshold:

There are four corners to her bed,
Four angels at her head:
Matthew, Mark, Luke, and John;
God bless the bed she lies on.
New moon, new moon, God bless me,
God bless this house and family.

35: Amulet to Ward Off Lilith

ADAM AND EVE: LILITH, AVAUNT!
SINOI, SINSINOI, AND S-M-N-G-L-F.

Once upon a time, the prophet Elijah was walking along the road when he encountered the wicked Lilith accompanied by all her gang.

"Wither away, foul creature," he demanded, "thou and all thy foul gang?"

"Sir," she replied, "I am off to the house of Mistress X who is expecting a child. I am going to plunge her into the sleep of death, take away her babe, suck its blood, drain its marrow, and seal up its flesh."

"Nay," cried the prophet, "by the curse of God thou shalt be restrained and turned to dumb stone!"

"Not that!" implored the hag, "For God's sake, release me from that curse, and I will flee; and I will swear unto thee in the name of Jehovah, God of the armies of Israel, to forgo my intent against yon woman and her child. Moreover, whenever in future men recite my names, or I see them written up, neither I nor my gang shall have power to harm or hurt. And these be my names: *Lilith, Abitr Abito, Amorofo, Kkods, Ikpodo, Ayylo, Ptrota, Abnukta, Strina, Kle Ptuza, Tltoi Pritsâ.*"

36: Birth Customs from the Isle of Man

From the birth of a child, till after it was baptized, it was customary to keep in the room where the woman was confined, a *peck* or wooden hoop, about three or four inches deep, and about twenty inches in diameter, covered with a sheep's skin, and resembling the head of a drum, which was heaped with oaten cakes and cheese, of which all visitors may freely partake, and small pieces of cheese and bread, called *blithe meat,* were scattered in and about the house for the Fairies. The woman who carried the infant to church for baptism was also supplied with bread and cheese, to give to the first person she met on the way, in order to preserve her charge from evil influences. After returning from church, the remaining part of the day, and often a great part of the night, was spent in eating and drinking, to which "the whole country round" was invited, and they, in return, gave presents to the child. If, after childbirth, a woman did not recover her usual strength as soon as expected, she was then declared to be the victim of an "Evil Eye." Some neighbor is soon suspected of having given the envenomed glance; and to counteract its malignancy, a square piece was secretly cut out of some part of her garment, and burnt immediately under the nose of the afflicted woman. This was considered an infallible cure.

The baby, also, was supposed to be especially liable to be affected by the "Evil Eye" before baptism, and it was considered that the best way to prevent this was to keep it constantly within the same room in which it was born. Children were also supposed to be much more liable to abduction by Fairies before the same ceremony. From the time that a woman was delivered of a child, till thanksgiving for her safe recovery was offered up by some divine, or until the consecrated candle[1] — which was kept in her room at this time — was burnt, it was deemed

1. The churching of a woman, in the Manx language, is called *lostey-chainley,* from the practice of burning a candle, in former times, during this service.

requisite, as a protection for herself against the power of evil spirits, that she should keep her husband's trousers beside her in the bed, to prevent her infant being carried off by the Fairies, before being secured from their grasp by baptism. A person was invariably appointed for its special protection, and when she had occasion to leave the child in the cradle she would place the tongs, which must be made of iron, across it till her return.

Another specific to ward off evil from babies was to put salt in their mouths as soon as possible after their birth. In connection with this it may be noted that, as it was once the custom to expose infants in order that they might die, this practice may have been resorted to as a means of prevention. For, if the child had once partaken of any food, it could not be exposed. It was deemed most unlucky to cut their hair or nails before they were a year old, and, if it was done, the fragments were carefully burned. A posthumous child was supposed to have the gift of second sight, and the seventh son of a seventh son, and a child born on Halloween had powers of intercourse with the unseen world.

A child born with a caul—a thin membrane covering the head— would probably be notorious in some way. This caul was supposed to be a preventative against shipwreck and drowning, and was accordingly purchased by sailors. This idea of the value of a caul was widespread, as would appear from numerous advertisements in the newspapers. One of these, which appeared in the London *Times* in 1835, was as follows: "A child's Caul to be disposed of, a well-known preservative against drowning, &c., price 10 guineas." And a caul has been advertised for sale in a Liverpool paper in this year (1891).

—*A. W. Moore*

37: Signs, Lore, Omens from the United States

Some peckerwood folk in central Arkansas believe that if a husband sits on his roof for seven hours, near the chimney, his next child will be a boy. I have known several men to try this, but only one stuck it out for the full seven hours. He took a hammer up with him, and when anybody that he knew came along the road, he pretended to be fixing the roof. The next child *was* a boy, too.

—*Vance Randolph*

To dream of death is a sign of birth.
To dream about a fire means a girl friend is pregnant.
To dream of fish means you'll have a baby.
Every time a star shoots, a baby is born in that direction.

You will have as many children as the number of times the afterbirth
   pops in the fire when you burn it.
You will have as many children as the number of knots in the umbilical
   cord.

Hold a nickel in your mouth at conception and the child will be a boy.

If the man is sick during the first three months of his wife's pregnancy,
   the baby will be a boy. If the mother is sick during this time, the baby
   will be a girl.

—*Ray B. Browne*

If you carry the baby low, it'll be a boy.
If you carry the baby high, it'll be a girl.

If you're pointed, it's a girl.
If you're round or broad, it's a boy.

If he's active, it'll be a boy.
If he's calm, it'll be a girl.

Swing a silver needle over the mother to tell if it's a boy or girl.
Swing a golden ring over the mother to tell if it's a boy or girl.
If it spins, it'll be a girl.
If it swings, it'll be a boy.

—collected by Lucile F. Newman

He who is born on New Year's morn
Will have his own way sure as you're born.

He who is born on Easter morn
Shall never know want, or care, or harm.

A child born on a saint's day must bear the saint's name.
It is unlucky to take away the day from it.

—collected by Fanny D. Bergen

An open hand in a baby is a sign of a generous disposition, but a habit of
closing the fingers indicates avarice, or, as we say, closefistedness.
A double crown on the head means that the owner will "break bread in
two kingdoms."
A child born with a silver veil over its face will never be drowned. Many
sailors are known to wear the caul with which they were born about
their person as a charm against death by drowning.
If a child cries at birth and lifts up one hand, he is born to command.
If the baby smiles in its sleep, it is talking with angels.
A child born with two cowlicks will be bright.
If you preserve the umbilical cord your child will become bright and
clever.
A child born with long hair will not live long unless it soon falls out.
A child born with teeth won't live long.
If a child is born on the first day of a zodiacal sign, the next child to be
born will be of the same sex. If however the sign of the zodiac changes,
the sex of the following child will also change.

Bad children are born under an evil star.
A person born in January can see ghosts.
A child born on April 1 will not live long.
A child born in Libra will have skin diseases.
A child born in the sign of Leo will become strong.
Lucky the child born in Virgo.
A child born in the sign of the Crab will not prosper or it will decline.
Any born in the sign of Taurus will be stubborn.
A man born in the sign of Pisces is always thirsty.
Unlucky the child born on the thirteenth of the month.
A child born on Sunday will be proud.
Anyone born on Wednesday will be stupid.
A child born on Saturday will be slovenly.
Children born on September 27th will be fond of women and strong
   drink.

Thursday has one lucky hour, just before sunset, for birth.

Monday's child is fair of face,
Tuesday's child is full of grace,
Wednesday's child is sour and sad,
Thursday's child is merry and glad,
Friday's child is loving and giving.
Saturday's child must work for a living;
But the child born on the Sabbath Day
Is blithe and bonny and good and gay.
   —collected by Fanny D. Bergen and Edwin Miller Fogel

If a woman leaves a diaper under a bed in the home where she is visiting,
there soon will be another birth at that house. Hence the sayings: "Don't
leave a diaper here"—when the hostess does not desire a child; and,
"Somebody left a diaper"—after a child has been born.

   A woman on the first visit to a newly born child should not hold it in
her arms, for she will become a mother.

   If a married woman is the first person to see a recently born infant, she
will have the next child.

   The woman who lays her coat or hat on a strange bed will get a baby.

   If outgrown baby clothes are given away the mother will soon need
them again.

To find a baby's pacifier means an approaching birth in the family.

The itching of a woman's loins is the sign of a birth.

"If there are three women sitting in a room and all three are menstruating, it is the sign that one of them will be pregnant before the year is out. I was sitting in a room with two ladies and all three of us were menstruating. I laughed and said, 'It won't be me being pregnant, for I have been married eighteen years and have no children'. They had the laugh on me, for before the year was out I was pregnant and the only child I have was born."

"Some people say that if a couple gets married and go to a picture show within the first three days they will have twins."

"They say that if you go swimming the first day you are married you will have twins."

A bright star in the sky indicates that there will soon be a birth.

A woman will soon have a baby, if she dreams that her mother has had a child. One woman before the birth of each of her four children dreamed that her mother had had a child.

Dreaming of a baby foretells another child coming into the family.

Count apple seeds to discover the number of your future children.

Blow a dandelion seed ball and the number of seeds left will show how many children you are going to have.

The number of knots or lumps on the navel cord of the first baby reveals how many children will be born to the mother.

If you want to learn the number of your future children, attach a wedding ring to a string and lower it into a glass tumbler, and ask, "How many children shall I have?" The ring will answer by swinging to and fro against the sides of the glass, and each distinct strike signifies one child.

Count the veins branching out from the main vein in your wrist and that will be the number of children you are going to have.

Count the wrinkles in your forehead and you will know the number of your future children.

A poor man is certain to have many children.

Children of late marriages are unhealthy and short-lived.

A happily married couple will procreate good-looking children. If a husband and wife quarrel continually, their children will be ugly.

Twins run in every third generation.

If a man and his wife couple twice at the time of conception, they will have twins; if three times, then triplets.

Children conceived while the father or mother, or both, is intoxicated will be idiotic or subject to epileptic fits.

The birth of a female proves that the woman is stronger than her husband.

When a male is born, the man has more strength than his wife.

"If you don't nurse your baby, you will soon have another."

While a woman is still nursing her baby, she will never be "caught." One woman said that she nursed her only child six years for this reason.

"Take a tablespoonful of bluing each morning for nine mornings. They say it will make you miscarry."

"If you want to miscarry, don't eat anything and take a half glass of sweet milk and two teaspoonfuls of black gunpowder. Take four doses four hours apart and it will bring you."

"If a woman that is pregnant will walk under a mare's neck at twelve o'clock noon for five days without touching its neck, it will make her miscarry."

"If you are pregnant, get on a horse and ride five miles just as hard as you can. If you don't lose it then, you will not."

"Take the water off rusty nails for nine days without drinking anything else and this will make you miscarry."

"If you will put nine rusty nails in some whiskey and senna tea and take it, it will sure make you miscarry. You may not live, but it will bring you."

"Take a half pint of vinegar and nine rusty nails and six tablespoonfuls of Epsom salts and let stand nine days before you take it. They say it will make you miscarry."

"Take ten cents worth of prickly ash, ten cents worth of senna leaves, one tablespoonful of store tea, and make a tea of each one. Then put them in a stone jar with a pint of whiskey and nine rusty nails. Let stand for nine days, then give a tablespoonful every two hours until they start to flow. It will make you miscarry. I know a woman that was seven months gone and she took this and she sure lost it."

"Make a tea out of peach leaves and the bark. Boil well and get it real strong and take. It will bring your sickness, if you are not over two months gone."

A miscarriage can be effected by taking fifteen grains of quinine.

Use senna tea for abortion.

Take turpentine once a month just before the period and impregnation will be impossible.

"If a woman gets in the family way during the change of life, no matter what she does she cannot get rid of the baby unless she kills herself."

Boys are had more frequently by youthful than by elderly parents.

A woman whose right ovary has been excised can have females only.

Males only will be born to a woman after the removal of her left ovary.

When in coitus the woman's stimulation surpasses that of her husband's, a son will be conceived.

—Harry Middleton Hyatt

A mole on the neck,
You'll have money by the peck.
A mole on the ear,
You'll have money by the year.
A mole on the lip,
You're a little too flip.
A mole on your arm,
You'll never be harmed.
A mole on your back,
You'll have money by the sack.

Stay in the house and draw the curtains during an eclipse.

The moon and thunder are dangerous.

A full moon causes fights.

A Christmas Eve baby is a werewolf.

Garlic over the stomach wards off vampires.

I don't worry about such things because I wear a metal key at my waist to
protect the baby all the time.

—collected by Lucile F. Newman

It is common knowledge that in certain neurotic families the husband falls ill when the wife becomes pregnant. One man told me that his wife had six children, and that during each pregnancy he vomited every morning, and so on. The midwife confirmed his story, as did a local physician who was familiar with the case. This man's wife was much pleased, thinking that her husband's suffering indicated the depth of his affection for her and somehow made her pregnancy easier. "My man he allus does my pukin' for me," she told the neighbors proudly. Such a situation is not rare enough to cause much comment and is referred to as a sort of joke on the husband.

In Lawrence County, Missouri, a woman gave birth to a female child who was said to be "marked for a cat"—the mother having been startled by an unexpected encounter with a trapped wildcat in the fourth month of her pregnancy. This baby looked all right except that its body was unusually hairy, but it never learned to talk or walk erect. It mewed and growled like a cat, ate like a cat, and slept curled up on a pillow behind the stove. When the cat girl reached the age of thirteen she began to have "wild spells" at regular intervals, like an animal in heat. So the family built a stout cage outside the house, and shut her up while the "spell" lasted — a neighbor said that "you could hear her a-hollerin' and a-yowlin' half a mile off." I am told that this cat woman was still living near Aurora, Missouri, in 1941, and she must have been more than fifty years old at that time. In recent years, however, she has been very quiet. She sleeps most of the time and does not have to be caged any longer. I asked a physician who knew that neighborhood about the cat woman. "I have never seen this case," he answered, "but I have heard about her for many years. I don't doubt that they have got an idiot in that house, who walks on all fours, and is unable to talk. Doubtless she eats like an animal and behaves like one in other ways. You can see such creatures in any asylum. But all this stuff about her being 'marked' by a cat — that's just backwoods superstition. If the mother of that idiot had been scared by a wolf instead of a wildcat, the child would have been called a 'wolf girl,' and these farmers would imagine that the noises she makes sound exactly like a wolf growling."

Otto Ernest Rayburn, of Eureka Springs, Arkansas, tells of a woman who was frightened by cattle during her pregnancy, and the child had a strange cowlike face, "with two small growths protruding from the head like horns." Not only that, but the creature "emitted low, rumbling sounds like the bellowing of a bull!"

—Vance Randolph

Looking at bad sights marks the baby. Being scared by bad sights marks the baby.
Seeing dead people marks the baby.
Watching scary movies marks the baby.
If you look upon a monkey, your child will look like a monkey.
If you look at something like worms or snakes it will mark the baby.
A friend's husband was going with another lady who looked like a cow and when the baby was born she looked like a cow because she hated the lady.
My last baby has a gun mark on his back. He was marked because I wanted to take a gun to my husband.

I don't believe these things but I think you can't go wrong if you think good thoughts. I avoid watching science fiction movies and I read good books like the Bible and pray a lot. You should keep your mind on better things. I also play the piano a lot more.

—collected by Lucile F. Newman

If the cradle cap of a baby be combed with a fine-toothed comb, the child will be blind.

Hold a baby to a looking glass and he will die before he completes his first year.

If a baby yawns, the sign of the cross should be made over it so that evil spirits will not enter.

To rock the cradle when the baby is not in it will kill it.

One article of an unborn infant's wardrobe must be left unmade or unbought or the child is liable not to live.

Tickling a baby causes stuttering.

If an infant be measured, it will die before its growing time is over.

—collected by Fanny D. Bergen

IV Pregnancy

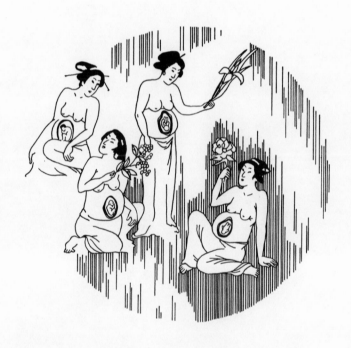

The romavali's thick stem supports
a pair of lotuses, her high and close-set breasts,
on which sit bees, the darkening nipples.
These flowers tell of treasure
hidden in my darling's belly.
                    —translated by Daniel H. H. Ingalls

38: Transformation Mysteries
of the Woman

The transformation mysteries of the woman are primarily blood transformation mysteries that lead her to the experience of her own creativity and produce a numinous impression on the man. This phenomenon has its roots in psychobiological development. The transformation from girl to woman is far more accentuated than the corresponding development from boy to man. Menstruation, the first blood-transformation mystery in woman, is in every respect a more important incident than the first emission of sperm in the male. The latter is seldom remembered, while the beginning of menstruation is everywhere rightly regarded as a fateful moment in the life of a woman.

Pregnancy is the second blood mystery. According to the primitive view, the embryo is built up from the blood, which, as the cessation of menstruation indicates, does not flow outward in the period of pregnancy. In pregnancy woman experiences a combination of the elementary and transformative characters.

The growth of the foetus already brings about a change of the woman's personality. But although the woman's transformation to motherhood is completed with birth, birth sets in motion a new archetypal constellation that reshapes the woman's life down to its very depths.

To nourish and protect, to keep warm and hold fast—these are the functions in which the elementary character of the feminine operates in relation to the child, and here again this relation is the basis of the woman's own transformation. Briffault looked upon the mother-child relationship and the female group behavior built upon it as the foundation of social life and hence of human culture. This well-supported hypothesis gains further cogency from the biological observation that the human species is the only one in which the infant, during the first year of life, may be regarded as an "embryo outside the womb." This implies that it completes its extrauterine embryonic life in a social environment essentially determined by the mother. This circumstance enhances the importance of the mother for the child and strengthens the mother's attachment to the child, whose embryonic dependency becomes a basis for her unconscious and conscious maternal solicitude.

After childbirth the woman's third blood mystery occurs: the transformation of blood into milk, which is the foundation for the primordial mysteries of food transformation.

— Erich Neumann

39: She Must Be Treated Like A Flower

A pregnant girl is supposed to get very *dhongi* (deceitful); she pretends to be in pain, demands attention, "craves" for a lot of things that she could be without. The husband has a very tender love for her at this time. "Even though she says, 'Don't leave me alone. Give me this to wear, that to eat. Stay with me all the time,' he is glad to do so for she is to be the mother of his child." "She must be treated like a flower, for otherwise the light may fade from her blossom."

—*Verrier Elwin*

40: The Couvade

Couvade (derived from *couver*, to hatch) means "male childbed." In the case of a number of societies in transition, it has generally been considered one of the means by which the men take over the governing functions of the women. Roughly speaking, it means the following: When the woman gives birth, the man goes to bed sobbingly, writhes with ostensible pains, moans, has warm compresses applied to his body, has himself nursed attentively, and submits to dietary restrictions for days, weeks, or, in exceptional cases, even for months. Until his first bath afterward, he is considered unclean, just as though he had himself given birth to the child.

This custom, deviating widely according to the tribe in the time covered and other variables, was known very early, being mentioned by some of the famous travelers of antiquity. Herodotus lists its existence among certain African tribes. Nymphodorus attributes it to the Scythians at the Black Sea; Diodorus to the Corsicans; Strabo, to the Celto-Iberians of Spain, whose direct descendants, the Basques around the Pyrenees, practice it still. On the island of Cyprus, there used to be a couvade that was unconnected with any special birth: every year, at the festival of Aphrodite, a handsome youth had to lie down in an open tent and imitate by voice and emotions, a woman during her birth pangs. As for China, Marco Polo was the first European to report on couvades among the mountain tribe of the Miau-tse, and modern English explorers have confirmed his data.

The friendly zeal with which people are currently exploring, registering, and studying all exotic races photographically, phonographically, and photometrically in order to catch them before our indigestible civilization can ruin them and they disappear altogether has gradually uncovered the fact that the number of women writhing in childbed is not so much greater than that of men doing the same, that there has recently been, or still exists, a couvade in places from Siberia to South America, in the Malay Archipelago, in Africa, China, Brazil, and India, with cultured as well as uncultured races.

As obvious as the data seem, the meaning is obscure. There are as many opinions as there are scholars. Since customs are older than logic and have grown into our level as ancient hereditary property, the question about "reasons" is of little avail to those who ask it. Genuine customs exist and fade away within the zone of pure feeling, without brushing the area of reason. Primitive nations, apart from their possible inability, dislike giving information about their actions, sense any suggestion of what the questioner wants to hear, and respond according to the unspoken wishes of their interlocutor. Could anybody ascertain in Germany or Switzerland today why a man's shirt is hanged in front of the prospective mother's window in Thuringia; or why in the canton of Aargau the woman dons her husband's trousers the first time that she leaves the house after the confinement; whereas in the Lech Valley she puts on his hat? No one in those places remembers what these customs are good for; the ethnologist, with his comparative data from five continents, says these are remnants of genuine couvades with their characteristic swapping of roles by the two sexes.

When the wife of a Brahman becomes pregnant, the husband stops chewing betel, which is more difficult than going without tobacco is for a smoker, and he fasts until she gives birth. In the Philippines, the father must stop eating sour fruit a week before the delivery; otherwise, the child will have a stomach ache. In Borneo, he is not allowed to use a cork; otherwise, the child will suffer from constipation. In China, the man must guard against violent movements or the embryo will suffer in the mother's body. For the same reason, the Jambim man abstains from fishing: the sea (great fecund water) is not to be stirred up by the beating of oars. The Malayans of the archipelago touch no sharp implements, kill no animals, and avoid any action that injures anything.

Before the babe is born, both parents are almost everywhere subject to strict dietary rules. But whereas the woman is usually permitted to move freely after the birth and, some food taboos apart, may resume a normal life, the man's postnatal couvade often begins at this point, with sadistic annoyances far exceeding the prenatal one. The Caribs of Cayenne make him lie in a hammock and fast for six months. Afterward, when he rises from it to return to his house for the first time, a mere skin and bones, the guests assembled there inflict bloody wounds on him with an aguti tooth and rub pepper into his bleeding sores. Really sick this time, he returns to his hammock and until the end of the seventh month eats neither fish nor fowl. La Borde relates that many Indian tribes of South America slash the skin of a young father after he has fasted a long time, left his hammock only at night, and been subjected to many other privations. Having inflicted bleeding gashes upon him, they then rub pepper and tobacco juice into them. He is not allowed to utter one cry in pain. His noble blood is then rubbed into the baby's face, so that it shall become as brave as he.

One can imagine what it would mean to be a father to suffer all these tortures in a polygamous society! Much of this maltreatment obviously belongs to the realm of sympathetic and imitative magic and is not an integral part of the couvade. Lucien Levy-Bruhl, and the entire French school of thought with him, thinks that these proceedings are only part of the precautionary measures and taboos that both parents impose upon themselves. The European only noticed them, especially in the case of the male because it seemed so unusual, and for this reason the couvade was analyzed as something apart from other birth rites, which had been a mistake. The "common fate," "mystical participation," "blood bonds" are, in his theory, so strong that whatever one person does is noticed and experienced by the other. That is why the Brazilian Bororo drinks the medicine where he buys it—in the pharmacy—if his child is sick in bed at home; for it is just as effective that way.

Thurnwald supposes that the real couvade is not a kind of make-believe but that the man actually feels the birth pangs. Tyler also concludes that it is sympathetic magic, which had always been considered a means in Ireland for transferring the birth pangs to the man. This is the much-discussed "transference of pain" discussed by Frazer. It was kept a well-guarded secret by the Celts. No scientist has ever been successful in watching it; we only know for certain that, if it is to be successful, the man must give his consent. The English observer Pennant tells us: "I saw the progeny of such a childbed come into this world gently, without causing his mother the slightest inconvenience, while her poor husband roared with pain in a strange, unnatural anguish."

In Estonia, every bride at her wedding gives her husband beer and rosemary to drink. She then crawls between the legs of the intoxicated bridegroom, which is supposed to transfer some of the birth pangs to him later on, if he does not wake up during the ceremony. Here, there is no consent, whereas the Celts consider it essential. According to Frazer, the birth pangs are not necessarily tranferred to the husband but may also be given to other men or to a wooden statue. Ploss and Bastian believed that the demons of puerperal fever were to be misled by the exchange of roles, confuse the man with the woman, and, after discovering their mistake, would be embarrassed and powerless. The Vaertings' theory is probably wrong: they thought the couvade was a survival of gynocracy, because the man, acting the part of the nurse, stayed in bed with the child to keep it warm, but this custom is practiced mostly below the equator.

Psychology, on the other hand, bases all the tortures and dietary restrictions on a father complex, with its traumas, commingled guilt complexes, fear of vengeance, tenderness, and hatred. Its entire reasoning concerning the couvade hinges on the well-known Freudian hypothesis of the patricide in the original horde, the mutual relinquishment of the desired mother by all the sons, and the establishment of the totem meal as a reminder of the eating of the father, "that remarkable event in human history which led to the formation of religion, art, and social organization."

Bachofen, who compiled countless examples of the couvade, settles on the *birth-giving* gesture of the man as the essential thing. He also regards the couvade as the father's attempt to a right to the child, though in a different sense from that of psychoanalysis. He sees in it a typical symptom of the transition from matriarchy to patriarchy. Actually, the couvade is found almost exclusively in matriarchal societies. "The father's masculinity subordinates itself to the female potential and reveals itself in maternal characteristics." The act of giving birth, then, still outweighs the act of procreation. Fatherhood alone is insufficient; only when the man has undergone the natural state of motherhood can he be a father.

Bachofen was the first person to include an analysis of adoption ceremonies in his discussion of the couvade. For instance, Zeus could not legitimize his illegitimate son Hercules until a goddess had performed the act of giving birth to him. "Hera mounted her bed, took Hercules to her body, and then let him drop to the ground along with her clothes, with which she mimed his true birth." A similar ceremony still accompanies the adoption ceremony among the matriarchal Dyaks of Borneo: the adopted mother climbs on a high chair in the presence of many guests and has the adopted child crawl backward through her legs. Medieval Europe, Arabia, and Byzantium had similar practices. The Abbot Guibert describes how Baldwin of Flanders was adopted by the duke of Edessa "according to the popular customs," that is, according to matriarchal laws: "He had the naked man step inside of his linen undergarment, embraced him, and affirmed the whole with a solemn kiss. The same was done by his wife."

A touchingly unselfish couvade is exercised by women who help their sons with their own bodies in overcoming the pains of puberty rites. These ceremonies are accounted the same as a rebirth. Through fasting, suffering, fainting, and trance the boy must recreate himself into a man. He endures the dangerous circumcision as well as a ritual of several months in the bush under the guidance of older men.

In Australia, where the women are badly suppressed, the acceptance of the son into male society means complete severance of relations with the mother. The mothers, therefore, are treated by the initiates "like persons in mourning and women in childbed at the same time. The women abstain from the same foods as their sons, who are enduring the circumcision far away in the bush; otherwise, he might be in danger. They rub down their bodies with oil or grease, which are considered medicinal in their effect. They live alone at fires separate from the tribal camp; no one may approach them or speak to them. Every morning before dawn, the mothers sing the prescribed songs. They sing while standing up, while waving burning logs in the direction where they presume the camp of the initiates to be. If one of the boys is freed from one of the dietary taboos, his mother seems also freed from it." (*Matthews.*) Never before was their mystical tie as strong as in the very period when the mother uses it for the last time as a last means of final separation. The paternal couvade wants to acquire a right to the child; the maternal couvade cedes it.

—Helen Diner

41: The Suffering of Birth

"I do not know how to observe the suffering of birth," said Shindormo. "Please instruct me how to meditate upon it." In answer, the Jetsun sang:

> My faithful patroness, I will
> Explain the suffering of birth.
>
> The wanderer in the Bardo plane
> Is the Alaya Consciousness.
> Driven by lust and hatred
> It enters a mother's womb.
>
> Therein it feels like a fish
> In a rock's crevice caught.
> Sleeping in blood and yellow fluid,
> It is pillowed in discharges;
> Crammed in filth, it suffers pain.
> A bad body from bad Karma's born.
> Though remembering past lives,
> It cannot say a single word.
> Now scorched by heat,
> Now frozen by the cold,
> In nine months it emerges
> From the womb in pain
> Excruciating, as if
> Pulled out gripped by pliers.
> When from the womb its head is squeezed, the pain
> Is like being thrown into a bramble pit.
> The tiny body on the mother's lap
> Feels like a sparrow grappled by a hawk.
> When from the baby's tender body
> The blood and filth are being cleansed,
> The pain is like being flayed alive.

When the umbilical cord is cut,
It feels as though the spine were severed.
When wrapped in the cradle it feels bound
By chains, imprisoned in a dungeon.

He who realizes not the truth of No-arising,
Never can escape from the dread pangs of birth.

There is no time to postpone devotion:
When one dies one's greatest need
Is the divine Dharma.
You should then exert yourself
To practice Buddha's teaching.

— Milarepa

42: Remedies

For morning sickness, crack a peach seed and get out the kernels. Beat them and make a tea from it.

An expectant mother should take Epsom salts every day to keep her bowels regular.

To stop vomiting during pregnancy, take one drop of chloroform in a glass of sweetened water.

43: The Full Moon Rises . . .

The full moon rises
Yet my head is clean
I go to the well
The full moon rises
The fish rejoice in the deep pool of Koeli-Kachhar
Branches of the mango grove bend low to the earth.

Moon of the second month casts its shadow
There is a new bud in the garden
My lord desires me for the scent of my flower.

Moon of the third month casts its shadow
The life within me desires strange food
I long for mud and kodon dirt.

Moon of the fourth month casts its shadow
With gifts my mother comes for Sidauri
I sit in her lap and eat the seven foods.

Moon of the fifth month casts its shadow
The secret life stirs within me
O my darling I can hear your heartbeats.

Who can tell what fish is in the deep water?
When they catch it, we will know if it is saur or kotri
Moon of the sixth month casts its shadow.

Moon of the seventh month casts its shadow
Black are my nipples — it will be my father
My belly is long — it will be my mother.

Moon of the eighth month casts its shadow
The hour approaches, my husband comes no more near me
I saw a snake in the path and it went away blinded.

Moon of the ninth month casts its shadow
How weary is the life within; when it sees its dark prison
It struggles to be free and make its camp on earth.
                    —translated by Verrier Elwin

44: Pregnancy Taboos

Having a baby has never been as easy as it might be—even for savage women. And yet we think of it as much less trying for them than for our civilized women. In making this comparison we entirely overlook all the social complications of the function, greater in savagery even than in civilization.

In primitive thought a woman is supposed to be able to influence the looks, health, character, and career of her unborn child in no end of ways. Consequently, great circumspection and self-deprivation are required of her. Diet is particularly important. Australians believe that congenital deformities are caused by the eating of forbidden things during pregnancy. A boy once told Roth that he was humpbacked because before his birth his mother had eaten porcupine. In the Islands of Torres Straits should an expectant mother eat *at,* a flat fish, or *gib,* a red fish, her baby would have poor eyes and an unshapely nose or be wrinkled like a dotard. To give him a good voice and lusty lungs she must eat certain kinds of shellfish which make a hissing sound while roasting. If he is born with a dark complexion, it means that his mother has been too lazy to roast the peculiar kind of earth eaten by women in pregnancy. In the Admiralty Islands a woman does not eat yams, lest her child be lanky, or taro bulbs, lest it be dumpy. Were she to eat pork, it would have bristles in place of hair. A Caffre woman does not eat buck or the underlip of a pig, lest her baby should be ugly or have a large underlip. Nor does a Thompson River Indian eat hare, lest he have a harelip. If a Thompson River woman ate or even touched with her hand porcupine or anything killed by an eagle or hawk, the child would look and act like them. If she ate foolhen or squirrel the child would be foolish or a crybaby. Among the Kabuis, a pregnant woman may not eat any animal that has died with young. In Serbia, if she eats pork or fish, her child will be cross-eyed or slow to talk.

In the islands of Amboina and Uliase, a pregnant woman is expected to restrain her appetite in general, otherwise her child will be greedy. In other ways maternal conduct is often of serious sympathetic import to the unborn. It is quite commonly believed, for example, that to ensure a safe delivery a woman should avoid all knots or ties or bands. Hence in some of the islands of the Malay Archipelago, she may not weave cloth or plait mats; nor, in parts of Germany, pass under a clothesline or spin or reel or twist anything. In the Uliase islands a woman is careful not to lean against a cooking pot, otherwise her child will be black. In Saxony, if she kicks a pig or hits a dog or a cat, the child will have bristles on its back or hair on its face. The superstitious Berliner believes that if she has a tooth pulled, her child will be born a cripple. Elsewhere in Germany a pregnant woman must beware of entering a court of justice or of taking an oath, otherwise her child will be involved for life in legal troubles. Should she pilfer, her child could not keep from stealing. Should she wear a soiled apron, touch dirty water, or pin on a nosegay, her child would be a coward or have ugly hands or a foul breath.

Likewise credulous of prenatal influences, many of our own country-women practice sympathetic magic for the good of an expected child. They surround themselves with beautiful objects that the child may have a love for the beautiful. They read poetry, listen to music, or look at pictures to endow the child with an "artistic temperament" or with poetical or musical tastes. One expectant mother I knew of hung a picture of a beautiful child where her eyes would often fall upon it in order that her own child might be beautiful.[1]

On the other hand, disfigurements or birthmarks are very commonly accounted for through "maternal impressions." Unwonted contacts with animals are often thought to be the cause of these experiences. We remember of course the necklace-hidden mark on the neck of Elsie Venner, and how she was supposed to have come by her serpent nature. Not far from the house chosen by Holmes for his heroine lives a man whose face was marked at birth with a great mole, from which now grows in the midst of his black beard an inch or more of grey hair, and his old mother says that when she was carrying him she was once hit in the same part of the face by a dead mouse flung out of the barn as she was passing.

During pregnancy a woman is peculiarly subject to devils or to black magic. She must therefore be on her guard. In some of the islands of the Malay Archipelago she never leaves the house without a knife to frighten

1. I have lately learned that the notion was not original with her. "Some mothers cannot fix their eyes on certain Pictures without leaving the complexion or some marks in their Infants." (*Decency in Conversation amongst Women*, p. 165. London, 1664.)

away evil spirits. In northern Celebes she must never go about with her hair down—flowing hair is ever a favorite lodging place for spirits. Basuto women wear a skin apron and Wataveta women, veils, to protect themselves against pregnancy witchcraft. The Estonian peasant should be careful to wear a different pair of shoes each week, to throw the devil off her track. The Nereids of Greece are malevolent to pregnant women. So women are expected to avoid their haunts, not to sit under plantains or poplars, not to linger near springs or streams. The Gypsy woman of Siebenburgen is careful to cover her mouth with her hand when she yawns, to keep the evil spirits from slipping down her throat—perhaps the original reason for this "form of politeness" under other circumstances.

Continence taboos during pregnancy are widespread. They are generally for the sake of the child. But they are sometimes for the sake of the woman and sometimes for her husband's sake. Her husband may be still further safeguarded. In the Caroline Islands his pregnant wife may not eat with him; in Fiji, she may not wait upon him. The Chinese husband did not see his wife at all during the latter part of her pregnancy. He sent twice a day to ask for her, to be sure, but "if he were moved and came himself to ask about her, she did not presume to see him." I have known American husbands who during this time were loathe to accompany their wives in public places, and if they went out walking with them at all, preferred to go after dark.

A pregnant woman has not only to think of herself and her family; it behooves her to be very conscientious in her relations to society at large. She can do so much harm if she is not careful. Among the Mosquito Indians, should she enter the hut in which an ill man is sometimes segregated, he would never recover. In Guiana if she eats game caught by hounds, they will never be able to hunt again. On the Amazon if she partakes of meat eaten by a domestic animal or by a man, the animal will die and the man will never be able to shoot that kind of game again. Among the Yakuts she causes the bullets of the hunter to misfire and the skill of the artisan to deteriorate. German peasants believe that were she to pass through a field or garden bed, nothing would grow in them for several years, or their products would spoil. Were she to enter a brewery, the beer would turn; a wine cellar, the wine would sour; a bakery, the bread would spoil.

Considering the dangers she is herself subject to and to which she subjects others, a pregnant woman is naturally more or less secluded. Among the Atjehs, should she have a visitor, she must take the precaution of not receiving him at once — to mislead the malicious spirits likely to have followed him into the house. Among the Gypsies it is not visitors, but moonlight, to which she must not be exposed. The Jewess of Bosnia or of Herzegovina never goes out alone at night. In the islands of the Malay Archipelago, a pregnant woman does not go out at night at all, or in Celebes, in the rain. The Yakuts do not allow her to eat at the table with others. Among the South Slavs, she may not attend public dances, and among the Pshaves she is excluded from all kinds of festivities. When a pregnant Wanderobbo woman goes visiting, she streaks her forehead with white clay. Out of doors the Jekri woman warns people off with a bell. In Central Africa, during her pregnancy a woman stays constantly indoors. Among some of the tribes of the West Coast, on the other hand, during the last three weeks of her pregnancy, she has to leave the village and live entirely by herself.

My grandmother tells me that in her day[2] women not uncommonly attempted to conceal their condition by lacing, and that in the latter part of pregnancy they rarely left the house, except perhaps for a short walk in the evening. Nowadays, fortunately, women are able to wear, if they wish, a disguise of loose instead of tight clothes, and they seem to take more exercise and to be more out of doors, but they are still apt not to receive guests or to "go into society." Their presence is supposed to be embarrassing to boys and girls and they are therefore expected to keep away from "young" parties. But there are many circles in this country in which they would also cause discomfiture to persons of any age. A woman whose husband had been in our diplomatic service in Europe once told me that having been in the habit abroad of dining out as long as she felt well, on her return to Washington she accepted a dinner invitation "without thinking." The result was so embarrassing to the other guests and consequently to herself that she dined thereafter at home. On a recent canoe trip on the upper Connecticut we stopped one midday at a farmhouse to buy eggs. All our overtures had to be carried on through a crack in the door, for, until the men in our party sauntered away, the mother of the six children playing around us and of an expected seventh was averse to meeting us.

— *Elsie Clewes Parsons*

2. And before. Many Gentlewomen — all the time of their going with child — wear long bellied, and strait laced garments.

V Birth

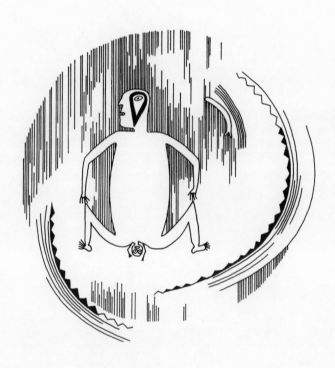

My heart is joyful,
My heart flies away, singing,
Under the trees of the forest,
Forest our home and our mother.
In my net I have caught
A little bird.
My heart is caught in the net,
In the net with the little bird.
          —translated by Willard R. Trask

45: Jicarilla Apache Birth Customs

A stake is driven into the ground, and the woman in childbirth kneels and clings to this. The stake is about three feet high, smoothed off so that she can hold on to it easily. Oak and other woods are used. Something, such as a hide, is placed beneath them.

A man, or another woman who is not menstruating, gets sick from smelling or touching the menstrual blood of a woman or the discharges at childbirth. This sickness comes out as rheumatism.[1] So the one who is taking care of the child at delivery always has to chew the root of "blood medicine" (*Bahia dissecta*) which has "blood" (red tendrils) at the ends of the roots. Otherwise, her hands will be knotted up; she'll have rheumatism through the knuckles and finger joints because she has to touch the child while it is still bloody.[2]

The head should come first in delivery. There is some belief about what causes a child to be born feet first. The mother has lain on something. When the child is caught and is not coming out right, or when the head is not coming first, the one who is taking care of the woman rubs her abdomen and back in an effort to get the baby out the right way. But internal manipulation is never attempted.

The child is not allowed to fall down. The midwife lifts it out and cuts the umbilical cord with a flint knife. She is careful not to cut the cord too short and she always ties it. They say that the navel will bleed and be sore if the cord is cut too short. After this, the first thing she does is to wipe the baby off. To make it cry, she shakes it, head up.

1. If, by any chance, a man does get rheumatism from such discharges, he is treated with a "blood medicine" (*Berlandiera lyrata*); "The leaves are cut off, boiled, and the liquid drunk. The medicine is also rubbed on the joints, and the seeds are chewed."
2. As this and other passages indicate, menstrual blood is considered to be one of the most dangerous and contaminating substances. Menstrual taboos will be summarized below. Sickness from menstrual blood resulted from the curse laid upon man by the daughters of a

Following the delivery, the mother blows four times on the hands of the midwife.[3]

> After this the midwife is safe; she could not get venereal disease even if she were with a man who had it, and she would not get the blood disease that gives you rheumatism either.

Prolonged and painful parturition may be considered a supernatural punishment. In one of the important traditional stories it is stated that

> . . . a woman who is kind and good does not suffer when she has a baby, but one who is mean and wicked and always harming others is the one who will have a hard time at childbirth.[4]

If labor is extremely difficult, careful external pressure may first be applied.

> Someone stands in back of the woman if the birth is not easy, putting her arms around her so that they cross in front high on the body, just below the breast. Then she runs her hands down slowly, pressing gently. This moves the baby down and it comes out.

Should such means fail, herbalism is likely to be tried next. The woman may be given a root called "medicine for birth" to chew, or she may take one seed of bird's-foot trefoil. A decoction made from a buffalo bezoar is said to hasten a long-delayed delivery.

> If a woman has been in labor for about three days, and the baby has not come, some of this stone is chopped up and boiled. She drinks the liquid, and the baby comes quickly.

But usually ceremonialists, men or women, are called in at such times.

> When labor is difficult, a ceremony is conducted over the woman. A man may conduct it. The horse ceremony is used a great deal for this purpose, because a mare has such an easy time bearing her young.[5]
>
> Sometimes the bowstring is used in a ceremony, because it is thought that the baby is being kept back by the umbilical cord which is wrapped around its

---

monster when they were sexually rebuffed by the culture hero. See Opler, *Myths and Tales of the Jicarilla Apache Indians*, p. 67.

3. Four is the Jicarilla sacred number and appears constantly in ceremonial contexts. Occasionally multiples of four are used.

4. Opler, *Myths and Tales of the Jicarilla Apache Indians*, p. 69.

5. The importance of the horse in Jicarilla culture can be judged from the many ways in which it is introduced into ceremonialism. In speaking of his need for horses one Jicarilla explains: "Some of us, when we go out hunting, have to carry in the deer on our backs. When we move, some of us who need more horses have to carry heavy loads on our backs. Some people are very poor and need more horses. If we had enough horses we could hunt deer easily in the mountains, load the meat on the horses, and come home with it quickly." (Opler, *Dirty Boy*, p. 7.)

head and neck. The one who conducts this ceremony takes the bowstring from the bow and motions with it along her body, from head to foot. This stands for the umbilical cord.[6]

As soon as the infant is born, someone hastens to put a blanket over the entrance to the dwelling to keep out the sun and the wind—the sun for the protection of the child, who "has tender flesh and might be harmed" by exposure to its rays before four days have elapsed; the wind for the sake of the mother, whom "it will kill at once if it gets in her; the wind is very bad for a woman when she has just had a baby."

At the very moment of birth there begins for the child a process of identification with persons and forces that will care for him throughout life.

> Both ears are pierced as soon as a baby is born. The grandmother (either the mother's mother or the father's mother) does it. If no grandmother is living, a mother's sister or a father's sister can do it. It must be done by a woman. A thorn is used to make the holes. It is done so that those things that watch over the Jicarilla will recognize the child and help him. Without this he will not be listened to or helped.[7]

The afterbirth is sometimes buried, sometimes burned, but the preferred mode of disposal is to place it in the top of a small Douglas spruce.[8] "The idea is that as the tree grows, so will the child."

Special attention is given the umbilical cord.

> It is never thrown away, but is always kept by the mother. She takes it wherever she goes. If a mother threw it away or disposed of it, her child would die.
>
> When a mother dies in childbirth, the cord is kept by a grandmother, a mother's sister, or some other close female relative of the child and the mother. If the mother dies after keeping the cord for many years, it is put on a young Douglas spruce.

Despite the fact that multiple births and certain types of abnormalities are considered supernatural punishment, there is no socially sanctioned infanticide.

> We keep deformed children and twins. If a child is born deformed, it is because the mother looked at the dancers while she was carrying the child, or

6. Note that once more a string, this time the bowstring, symbolizes the umbilical cord. There is a general association between lengths of buckskin or sinew, sunbeams, spider thread, and the umbilical cord.
7. In view of the meaning of this act, it is interesting that the grandparent, who is, as we shall see, the accepted instructor of the grandchild, is the one who performs it.
8. Associating a child with a growing tree, usually a Douglas spruce, to assure health and longevity, is common in Jicarilla culture. Another instance of this is found immediately below.

perhaps at a crippled or deformed person. If a baby is born dead, it happened either because the woman worked too hard or because she hurt the child to get rid of it.

Twins come if a woman forgets and sleeps on some men's clothing. There is no special way that twins are treated. But twins, whether of the same sex or a boy and girl, have one life together. If one twin dies, the other will soon die or will have a short life. Twins are considered two different people, though.

Sometimes unmarried mothers throw their babies away. But there is a strong feeling against it. To kill a child like this is to set yourself against life, and your own life will not be long after that.

The new mother pays strict attention to her health, her diet, and the feeding of her child immediately after the birth.

After childbirth a woman should rest up. She shouldn't start working right away. She wears a belt to keep her abdomen in and continues to wear it until she is in shape again. As soon as the blood stops coming, the woman is up and around again. She is told to drink a lot of soup so that she will have plenty of milk for the baby. She eats dried meat only; to do otherwise would make both mother and baby sick. She is not supposed to eat fresh meat until she is good and strong again.

The child is given water at first, for sometimes the mother has no milk yet. They feed the child soup or water for the first two days, until the mother's milk is proper. Or if another woman has milk, they let this woman feed the child till the mother is ready. If the mother has no milk at first, she just keeps nursing the baby till the good milk comes. But if she has no milk at all, they get another woman whose baby has died to nurse it.

While the mother is nursing the child, she should not eat tongue, lest the child be slow in learning to talk. She cannot eat chili either, or the child will have a bad stomach ache all the time. The mother has to be very careful what she eats when she is feeding the child.

If the mother's milk is not flowing well, and the child is sickly because of it, an old woman, a relative, will suckle the mother, will clean out her breasts. She does not swallow the milk, but spits it out on the ground. Then, when the mother is well again and the milk is flowing freely, the baby is given the breast once more.

For women who do not regain their health speedily following childbirth, a number of remedies, most of them herbal, may be prepared. Leaves of watercress are boiled for about two hours, and the liquid is drunk three times a day. The roots of *Eriogonum racemosum* are pounded and boiled and the liquid drunk. Sometimes alum root is mixed with this medicine. Cinquefoil roots are prepared and taken the same way. Anglepod seeds and leaves are boiled, and the resulting medicine is rubbed on if the joints ache. The same decoction may be used on a baby that is ill and feverish. Boiled roots and tops of *Bahia dissecta* yield a medicine to be taken internally and also rubbed on the body after childbirth.

Eriogonum jamesii is used for complications following a birth.

The roots, leaves, and flowers are pounded and boiled. The liquid is drunk twice a day by women after childbirth so that the blood will come out. The woman rubs her joints with the water too.

The leaves of the New Mexico rubber plant serve a similar purpose.

If the blood does not come out after delivery of the child, the woman is given "coffee" made from the leaves. She drinks it until the blood all comes out easily.

Juniper needles or the seed pod and flower of arrowhead are crushed and taken in water for the same trouble, or a "tea" made from monkey flower or puccoon may be given.

If, on the other hand, a woman bleeds excessively following delivery, she drinks each morning a medicine made from the boiled stems of Mormon tea. Liquid from the pounded and boiled roots of *Androsace pinetorum* or of wild geranium is also recommended for this trouble. The crushed root of the former may be rubbed on the abdomen, and the root of the latter is sometimes chewed fresh. By some, the egg of the black phoebe is considered as efficacious as any plant.

It is used by the woman whose stomach remains enlarged and who has blood and matter coming out of the vagina after it should have stopped. The egg is broken in water and boiled and the liquid drunk. This is done each morning till the condition gets better.

For a continuing pain in the lower dorsal region following childbirth, a plant belonging to the chickweed family is pounded and put in hot water; "then the patient's back is cut with flint till the blood flows, and the medicine is rubbed on."

For sore breasts, redtop is recommended: "If a woman's breasts are so sore and enlarged that she cannot nurse her baby, this grass is burned and the ashes put on them." But, "if a woman's baby dies and her breasts hurt, she works them with her hands and makes the milk come out to relieve herself."

—Morris Edward Opler

46: Haitian Birth Customs

The love of children, and the prestige which a man gains as head of a large family, are factors that go far to explain the desire for numerous progeny. In this not only is he aided by his own sophistication in matters of sex — for in Haitian peasant culture, one encounters no such conventionalized naïveté as the ignorance of physiological paternity found in certain other, non-African societies — but his desire is furthered as well by the absence of contraceptives and the emphasis laid by the Church, State, and African tradition on the desirability of many offspring. Though situations do arise when, because of illicit relations between a man and woman that result in conception, an abortion is held necessary, usually as soon as a woman discovers that she has conceived, she proceeds to take the necessary protective measures. First she goes to the old women of her own family, who give her herbs for the "three baths" she must take on each of the three succeeding days. This accomplished, she next visits a priest or priestess of the *vodun* cult who has the confidence of her family or of her husband's, and procures other herbs also for the purpose of preparing baths, and, in addition, a magic charm to wear about her neck or about her waist. This charm protects both herself and the child in her womb against the evil eye or any other evil spirit or evil magic that may be directed against her. If she is a worshipper of the African deities of the *vodun* cult, she may also ask the *vodun* priest to determine by divination what spirit will protect the child, and what her own deity asks to insure his aid. During all her pregnancy she is particularly careful to avoid eating those foods which are "hateful" to her — that is, which cause her to become ill — though in Mirebalais, at least, it is not necessary that she refrain from partaking of the foods "hateful" to her husband. A pregnant woman has privileges and powers not shared with other women, as was evidenced when a Haitian man once appeared with his eye half shut, explaining that the sty was a punishment for his refusal to buy something his pregnant spouse had coveted. "They do not always know they are sending you a sty, but it is a power they have," he made clear.

Shortly before parturition is expected, both the pregnant woman and her husband invoke the aid of the family deities and make them offerings of a *couvert sec*. The rite is an informal one that need not necessarily take place in the familial house of worship; if it is more convenient, it may be performed inside their own house or in the courtyard. After repeating the Pater Noster and the Ave Maria, a prayer such as the following is pronounced by the woman:

> *Toutes mystères, tant pour papa que manman, du même de côté mari moin: m'ap mandé ou pou' moin fait un heureuse accouchement, pou' l'ouv'i chemin ba moin.* — All the gods, both of my father and of my mother, as well as those of my husband: I ask that you cause me to have a good delivery, that you open the road for me.

At the same time the family ancestors are not overlooked:

> *Moin mandé nou' tous pou' nou' vini délivré moin, pou' nou' l'ouvri chemin pou' moin, pou' pas quitté malin esprit barré chemin qu'en moment delivrance moin apé' rivé. Nou' toutes Invisibles, les Saints, les Morts, Marassa, vini assité moin jou'a.* — I ask you all to come deliver me, that you open the way for me, that you do not allow evil spirits to bar my path when the time of the delivery approaches. May you all, Invisible Beings, the Saints, the Dead, Twins, come to my aid on that day.

Should one of the couple be a devotee of Damballa or Erzilie, both of them jealous gods, a chicken or two is added to the customary offerings, and some gift pleasing to the god, such as a dress or suit of his sacred color, is made him. Normally no further precautions need to be taken. If, however, the pregnant woman has had one or two miscarriages, she and her husband go to a *vodun* priest, preferably a woman, and obtain a "medicine" to be used in bathing the abdominal and vaginal areas as a precaution against *mauvaises aires,* the werewolves believed to consume children in the womb. If the pregnancy this time terminates successfully, some of the same medicine is rubbed on the child shortly after birth and several times during the ensuing weeks, but should the infant later fall ill, the *vodun* priest brings herbs and makes a smoke-fire to drive away the werewolves that are believed still to be hovering about.

At the onset of labor, if either the father or the mother of the unborn child is vowed to Damballa, another sacrifice is made to this god and to the spirits of twins, giving a *couvert sec* and one or two chickens and pigeons to each. If a *vodun* priest has determined what deity protects the child, a sacrifice is also given this spirit, and prayers are said to the spirits of twins, the dead of the families of both the man and the woman, and all other supernatural beings, saints, of the Church and *vodun* gods alike.

Meanwhile the woman has been placed on the ground on a mat or a cloth, supported in a reclining position with pillows and cloths, or on a covered box standing about a foot from the ground, with her legs drawn up. No fire is built in the house, all doors and windows are tightly shut, and covers are provided against a chill. A candle stands lighted at the threshold, and holy water is poured beside it; a candle is also often lighted in the church before the statue of the saint who corresponds to the *vodun* deity under whose protection the woman in labor is thought to be. In the room with her is the midwife and as many as six, seven, eight, or nine older women belonging to the families of the woman and her husband. The hands of the woman are made to rest on her knees, but where labor is prolonged, her arms are supported above her head to afford relief. She is three times given very hot tea or a drink made of the stewed leaves of the mango tree and of the *bois lait*. The midwife, with palm oil on her hands, watches the rhythm of labor and presses on the abdomen to facilitate delivery.

If it becomes evident that this will be difficult, a *vodun* priest is at once called to determine by divination whether or not the deities who have been propitiated are satisfied. If the answer is a negative one, he promises future sacrifices or gives minor offerings immediately. Care is also taken to ascertain whether the trouble is due to the discontent of the family dead who may have been angered by neglect to wear mourning for them, or because sacrifices or a *service* due them have been delayed too long. Inquiries are similarly made to determine whether the spirits of twins might not be displeased, while the possibility that evil magic may have been invoked is not overlooked, especially if the husband has several wives. If the inquiry shows that the magic of a co-wife was responsible, a strong counter-charm is made at once. Should the woman in labor eventually die, however, her death is not considered to be the result of any act of infidelity on her part, and does not, as in other Negro cultures, prevent the usual burial and mourning customs being carried out.

The child is delivered on a mat or cloth placed on the ground, and the navel cord is cut with scissors, leaving a length of three finger breadths. The end of the cord is cauterized with a red-hot iron, treated with oil, and bandaged with a piece of cloth. If the infant emits no cry after birth, the midwife shakes it or strikes it smartly to start its breathing, but should this be insufficient, a large *gammelle,* or wooden bowl used to serve food at feasts, is overturned so as to cover the child, and this is beaten for a few moments, a procedure which is held both to awaken the child and give it needed warmth. After being bathed in tepid water in which calabash leaves have been steeped, about a teaspoonful of muscat, palm oil, and sugar is fed the infant. An abdominal band is put on in place, and the child is dressed in a nightgown tightly pinned, so as to envelop its form and cause it to grow straight-limbed and firm of muscle. The process of moulding the head is begun at once, pressure being applied once a day for the first three days of life. The nostrils are pinched every few moments during the first day of life and several times each of the succeeding days, to cause them to be narrow. This matter of shaping the head and compressing the nostrils is sufficiently important to have figured in the accounts of birth conventions as given by a number of persons, though there is some disagreement as to the details of the practice, some maintaining that the head is shaped every eight days for two months and the nostrils compressed many times a day for a period of eight days. The baby continues to be bathed in tepid water, and, if born during the winter months, a fire always burns in the house.

The placenta is buried in a special hole dug in the room where the birth occurred, the preferred places for this being beneath the bed or at the threshold. Any of the women in attendance may bury the placenta, though usually the midwife sees to its disposal. If delivery takes place during the day, it is buried immediately after ejection, but if the birth has occurred during the night, they wait for daylight. Salt is added to the hole, "so that the evil eye cannot take it (for magic purposes), for with salt it spoils very quickly." Neither the hole nor its contents are held to be of future importance, and though the child may be shown where the cord and placenta were buried, by that time nothing will remain of it which might be of use to a maker of charms. After three or four days the cord falls off and muscat powder is applied to heal the wound cleanly. The bit of cord is saved, and if the child becomes ill, this is boiled and the water given as a drink. Occasionally an entire umbilical cord is dried and retained; and one woman spoke of the cord of her mother as still being in existence.

The mother is also bathed in water in which calabash leaves and other ingredients have been steeped, and after being carefully dried, a band is tightly tied about her abdomen to give her support. A cloth is placed to cover the vagina, which is not cleansed until the following day, though after that the vaginal region is washed twice daily for some forty days.

Red wine is given to women immediately after delivery to sustain them until food can be prepared. Bananas, salt fish, milk, chocolate, and a dish of stew made of chicken and rice are offered, and in most instances the women eat heartily.

The cloths used during childbirth are carefully guarded, the woman herself or a trusted member of her family seeing to the task of washing them, so as to prevent their being used for evil magic. If a miscarriage occurs, the fetus is buried in a hole dug in the floor of the woman's house while the woman herself is bathed and otherwise cared for as in the case of a normal delivery.

A woman is usually up and about three or four days after the birth of her child, or sooner if there is no one to help her with her household duties, in which case she may even be obliged to perform the heavy work of going to the river for water within the week, though she is careful not to bend down or to get her feet wet. When possible, however, she waits for from fifteen to twenty days before doing this kind of work, and, in any event, she will not bathe in cold water until more than a month has passed. A week or two after giving birth she may resume her selling in the market, and two months after her child is born she will take up work in her garden.

During this period of the mother's recovery, the child is ritually introduced to his world and to the spirits which govern it. Three or four days after the cord drops, the midwife, water and a candle in hand, presents the child to the sun and the four corners of the earth, speaking an invocation which none but women of this profession may know or hear spoken. The child is then carried into the courtyard before the house, though he may not be taken elsewhere for as many as three weeks. When he is taken across the threshold for the first time, he is cradled in the left arm of the one who carries him; in the left hand water is held, while the right hand holds a lighted candle. Water is thrown in three directions, outward from the door and to each side of it, as the child is taken about the outside of the house. This rite is repeated by everyone present at the time, but water is "thrown" only once.

Though it is said by some that a child is not given a charm immediately after birth unless it is ill, it is nevertheless customary to place a cord about the neck of an infant on the day it is born, to remain there until some three or four years later, when it wears out and is lost. There is no difference of opinion, however, on the point that if a baby falls ill soon after birth, steps must be taken to give it spiritual protection. A *vodun* priest is called to make a charm for it to wear, while, in addition, another

112

charm is placed in the house to guard its inhabitants against "all bad things," such as the evil eye — since this tends to give babies convulsions — demons, werewolves, or the "little folk" who bring bad magic. A *jok* against harm resulting from even unconscious envy is also provided, since an individual who admires a baby because of its good health or good looks or some other attribute may unwittingly bring harm to it. For such reasons the child is often burned slightly on the cheek, a ritual carried out by the *vodun* priest in order that the scar may "give one with evil intentions toward the child an 'occupation' to divert his attention, that would otherwise be devoted to carrying out some evil design."

There is some question as to whether, as in so many Negro cultures, the child is given a special name at birth which is regarded as sacred and a thing to be concealed. In one instance it was stated that while one's "real" name was that given at the time of the Church baptism, everyone has a "nickname" *(petit nom)* that is known to the father and mother alone until the child is old enough to guard its secret character. This name is never spoken aloud, for if an enemy came to know it, he might use it for purposes of black magic against its owner. However, no agreement exists in Mirebalais as to this practice, which may represent a survival of a widespread West African custom.

A child born with a caul is believed to be "strong" in combating all evil spirits. The caul is dried and reduced to powder, and the infant is given some of the powder in water two or three days after birth. If a child is born with the navel cord wrapped about his throat, he is believed by some to be destined for leadership, though others do not hold this to be a significant omen. A child born feet-foremost is regarded with distaste, so that were it possible, he is turned about in the womb to facilitate a head presentation. If this cannot be done, the child when he grows up is reproached: "You came like a demon." More often, however, if a child with breech presentation is not stillborn, it is not believed that he will long survive. All such occurrences are attributed to bad magic, and the husband does not delay to seek out a diviner to discover for him what supernatural forces had caused the evil.

Breast-feeding begins on the third day, but if the milk does not come, the mother goes to a woman "specialist" who knows the herbs which are believed to induce the flow. When the mother is ill or tubercular, the infant is given a wet-nurse. Once he has begun to nurse, he is fed whenever he cries, and as soon as he can sit up he is given the same food as the mother eats. For the first two or three months after the birth of her child a woman refrains from eating eggplant, fresh fish — although she may eat salt fish—white beans or any others larger than Congo peas, pork, lard, and all fruit. The ears of a female child are pierced when she is about a month old for the gold earrings which are worn by girls and women of all ages. If the parents cannot afford them at that time, however, thread is placed in the holes until a sum sufficient to provide this important trinket has been accumulated.

—Melville J. Herskovits

47: The Birth of Dūan and Song's Baby

Dūan and her husband, Song, had a two-year-old son, Chaī. They lived and worked with her widowed mother, Lek, and her unmarried sister, Mī. The comfortable house stood high on piles, surrounded by rice fields. On a nearby mound lived Saī, sixty years old and full of energy, the youngest sister of her grandmother.

Now Dūan noticed that again her menses had stopped. Her mother had described before her marriage what this meant. With happiness in her eyes, as the first time, she told her husband, then her mother, and at the first opportunity, her husband's parents. There was no reason to keep her pregnancy secret. Since she and Song would be happy to have either a boy or a girl, she did not seek out the ritual means which existed to induce a child of a particular sex.

During the months of anticipation, Dūan worked along as usual in farming and housekeeping. Lek reminded her of prudent behavior. "Women are easily upset when pregnant. It is up to you to put yourself in a cheerful mood. Everything you do will affect the infant in your womb. If you see a scarred person, your child will be scarred. Be calm, look only at pleasant things and avoid jerky motions. Do not overeat, lest the child be a glutton. If you sleep during the day and are inactive, you will also have a lazy child. Some girls are trying to be like Bangkok people, pleading that they cannot do heavy work in the last few weeks of pregnancy, but that will cause a difficult labor."

To increase her appetite, early in her pregnancy Dūan visited a Chinese pharmacist to get medicine. He had so many kinds she hardly knew which to choose. He also had all-purpose kits for mother and baby, even one with fourteen different kinds of medicine "to control the body's temperature and keep the organs functioning." She decided on one of the favorites, pickled medicine (*jaa dauaung*), and from then on took a spoonful twice a day. She avoided all peppery-hot foods which would "damage the delicate complexion of the infant in the womb, burn off its hair, and maybe even kill it." Some women said they craved sweet, hot, or sour foods, but Dūan did not. A friend who had never eaten cobra curry so longed for its hot taste during her pregnancy that her mother gave her a small dish. She could not resist secretly finishing the whole pot! What heat and sleeplessness! To cool herself, she had sat in the canal. The baby, saved only because its mother drank the water from a young coconut fruit, "could resist the cobra heat because it was six months along, but even so, it shed its skin at birth." But another woman, pregnant seven months with her third child, also craved cobra curry, ate a lot, and said she did not feel hot. Nothing at all happened! The second woman was nearer to delivery, so stood the heat better, but more important, each individual was different. Because of Karma, of virtue and sin in former lives, each woman—and man, too—was born under different astral confluences and had lived and suffered differently.

About the seventh month, Dūan pondered who should help her at her delivery. Some of her friends were delivered by their own mothers, but Lek had undertaken the delivery of another daughter's child, and the baby had died in an hour. Because of this precedent of misfortune, Dūan suspected that her mother, therefore, would prefer not to do it, and knew that she herself would feel uneasy. So she decided for safety's sake to ask a midwife. She and Song could well afford the ceremonial offering with its customary twenty or so *baht,* even though the midwife said it was "as you please." A great many women never consulted with a midwife beforehand at all, but just sent word to the nearest one when the pains started or when trouble was encountered. Midwives varied in their capabilities, however, and Dūan wanted not only a good one but someone she knew well. Muslim midwives were said to be skilled, but they happened to live too far from her. Dūan decided to ask her elder aunt, Saī, who was a well-known midwife. Everything was right about Saī. She had experienced hands, a true desire to help, and effective magic; and she was a relative. Best of all, her own babies had eaten and slept well, had cried little, and now were grown to maturity. With such proof of merit, capabilities, and fortunate relations with supernatural powers, what better person to help Dūan start her baby on its earthly existence? Actually, if something happened, and Saī could not come, Dūan knew she would not be alone or unassisted. Almost every woman, and quite a few men, had seen childbirth not once, but many times, so willing hands abounded. So, one day, Dūan went to Saī. "Will you help me, and come when I call you? Please do not go far at that time." Saī agreed, knowing in her heart she had expected to care for Dūan. No day could be calculated because the baby decided when to be born. Dūan came home very fast, for doing so would help ensure a fast delivery.

As the weeks passed, Song, the new child's father, collected outside the house a great cone of *sakāe* firewood from their land. This wood was for the postpartum fire beside which Dūan would lie for many days. As the fire had to be very hot, a great deal of wood was needed, all to be collected beforehand. Song also covered the outside of the pile with thorny woods to keep away evil spirits. On her part, Dūan knew that everything needed for delivery was ready in the house as part of the regular household staples or utensils. Nothing need be bought except possibly a little Borneo camphor to mix with lemon grass for faintness, and alum. The midwife should never bring anything with her because it was essential to use what was in the house. Anything lacking could be quickly borrowed after the pains started. The little cushion on which the baby was to lie was cut, and half-filled with kapok. It was not sewn up, lest it induce by example a closed-up exit from the womb, or suggest a malplaced or deformed baby which had to be delivered onto a pillow. No one wanted to prepare for such an unhappy event. No clothing was bought for the child ahead of time for then the child might die, and all would have to be destroyed.

Dūan felt at ease and yet somewhat frightened at the prospect of the pain ahead. At an ordination she attended one night she listened again to the chant she had heard many times:

> In childbirth a woman has pain all over her body. . . . She is losing her soul and feels so frightened, despairing, and suffering that she throws herself up and down from time to time as if her mind were terribly wounded by the poisonous arrow of a hunter. She is uneasy and moans loudly as if a big mountain had fallen down upon her, and she is supposed to wait for death. She does not recover even if massaged by someone. She does not think of her pain, but tries to save the child's life, when, after the pushing wind comes, he is born.

On other occasions she pondered the deep satisfaction of her maternal role, then laughed in recalling a crafty woman who "faked labor pains to hold down her errant husband!" or so a sour mother-in-law said.

Finally, one day, Dūan felt uncomfortable and decided not to go out to plow. Lek prepared for her hot-tasting medicine. When Song came in at eleven from work, he went to the garden, to the little house of the family's protecting spirit (*sān phra phūm*), lighted incense and offered flowers, asking that it help his wife and keep away evil ghosts. He also prayed for help of the ancestors. Mī went to ask Saī not to go far away that day and to ask in what exact direction to push over the woodpile. Saī replied, "Push it over in the direction the Snake lies today, so that Dūan and the wood lie parallel with her head and its apex in the same direction to the north and east. Never let them be to the south and west." A passing boatman saw the wood go over. "There's news to tell!" he said. "The child is being born!" Dūan thought she ought to send away her little son, but he refused to go, and stayed by his mother the whole time. Song's sister came by for a visit, but stayed to help after getting word to their parents. It was no time for visitors, especially men, but any helpers, male or female, were welcome. Lek prepared the all-important ceremonial gift, the *khan khāo* (bowl-rice), for the midwife, which validated, and insured the use of, her private magic. She put a bunch of bananas, seven betel pepper leaves, seven areca nuts, flowers, incense sticks, a candle, and twenty *baht* into a bowl filled with dry rice grains. A little later she strung the holy thread around the four walls of the house. On each side she attached "*yan.*" These protective cloths, about ten inches square with magical letters and drawings, kept away the terrifying *phī krasū* spirits, seen as lights at night, who, attracted by bad smell and blood, would creep up the housepost and eat Dūan's blood, intestines, and feces through her anus. Then Mī went again to Saī to report that "the pain was increasing." These words were to signal to Saī that it was time for her to come.

As Dūan was to profit from the magic, it was better that she herself hand the midwife the *khan khāo* bowl. Saī lit the incense and offered the bowl in gratitude to the teacher who had given her her magic. She whispered in the direction of Dūan's head, "All good spirits in the high heavens and in the locality, help and do not obstruct at this delivery! Give happiness to mother and baby!" Placing the bowl on a high place to the side of Dūan's head, she said, "My teacher is long since dead, but will hear this request, and will pass the request and the *khan khāo* to her teacher, and so on, back all those thousands of generations, to the hermit Phra Khulīmān, who first discovered this magic. He got it from Phra In (Indra). He will make it good."

Dūan was sitting in the main part of the house. Her mother was seated behind her, arms under Dūan's arms, pressing down on the abdomen with every pain. She, Song, and others had taken turns thus supporting Dūan's back and pressing all afternoon. Dūan hoped it would not be like the first time when she had screamed with the pain of the tender spot where they constantly pushed. Their toes, digging into her thigh, also had left large bruises. Some women in the area had tried arm ropes, hung from the ceiling, on which to pull, and some women tried lying flat, but sitting while someone pressed was the usual way. Saī examined Dūan, and announced that labor was not very far along. She moved Dūan around so she faced another direction. "No wonder you are having a hard time," she said. "Your feet were pointing toward the *sān phra phūm* spirit house and you were not properly in line with today's direction of the celestial Prince-Snake (*Čhao Nāk*). By turning you thus, the baby will be born with, and not against, the scales that lie on the *nāk's* back. The Snake's direction differs each hour of the day, each day in the week, month, and season in the year. Today is Monday, so your head must be in the east, but Sundays, for instance, it must be to the north. You must also not face the Great Ghost (*phī lūang*).[1] Another being to respect is the *Čhao Krung Phā Lī*. Offerings to him must be at the feet or sides. If offered at the head, he would be angry at your disrespect, and you would have a fever and a terrible time. My grandfather taught me this from his Pali book. His was more accurate than the books in Thai one sees in the market."

Song was asked to boil up several kettles of water using this *sakāe* wood. Husbands always did that. "I was recently asked," said Saī, "to help at a woman's fourth child. I had been there for all the other three, and every time her husband was absent, gambling, I heard. He said he did not want to stay there because it was an awful sight. So it is, but there must be a man around: the husband; if he is dead, or gone, then a father or brother. I refused to accept that case because of the husband's neglect."

The winds that circulated in Dūan's body were not speeding fast enough to break the amniotic sac. Saī made her a medicine of *mung* bean and sugar, both of which wet the uterus, and murmured some magic words to help. Later she worked with her hands at the vagina, twisting the sac a bit to break it. Suddenly the sac ruptured.

Now the child was almost there. The head showed well. Saī sat down directly in front of Dūan to do the pressing herself. With one hand she held or gently pulled on the baby, with the other she pressed on the abdomen with every contraction. As she started in, she said magic words. She worked for an hour—no midwife would press more than that at a time—until at last the child was out. A little boy! With her finger Saī removed the blood from his mouth, and pucked out the lips. Breathing was slow in coming, so she shook him vigorously, then laid him down. Quickly she chewed up an onion and spit it over his body. "Ah-h-h!" A cry, though not very strong! Seeing the new baby appear, Chaī, who up to then had been constantly near his mother, rushed precipitously from the house, and refused to come in for hours, in spite of Song's and Lek's coaxing.

---

1. The Great Ghost makes a complete circle of all directions throughout twenty-four hours, and its direction of the moment must be avoided.

Everyone had observed an auspicious circumstance: the cord was looped around the baby's neck! This imitation of the holy cord (*mong-khon*) placed around head and neck in Brahman rites of passage was a rare and good sign. "A cord looped thus could never kill a baby," someone said.

Since the placenta was slow in coming, Saī prepared to cut the cord while Dūan rested and sipped the fiery snake brand medicine. Depending on circumstances she might cut it before or after the placenta was out. Taking a rhizome of *phlai,* a traditional healing root, she laid it on a clod of soil brought in from outside. From one of the old bamboo house beams, someone had sliced with a knife a sharp-edged, tapering sliver to serve as a cutter. The cord was stroked three times, starting near the baby's stomach "to remove the dirt." Then "something that is in the umbilical cord" was pushed back towards the baby's stomach "to prevent a flow of blood." She measured the cord from the baby's abdomen to his knee, and tied off two places in it with the holy unspun cotton cord used ordinarily in rituals. Laying the part between the two knots on the *phlai* on its bed of soil, and saying her magic: "*winyān a sam pa nō,*" she cut the cord with the bamboo cutter. With a chicken feather which had to come "from the mother's yard," she collected a few spider webs from the rafters, mixed them with coconut oil, and painted them around and on the cord-stump, also "to stop the blood-flow." While doing this, Saī said, "One midwife I know severs the cord by tying it with the thread at three places, then burns it with a flame."

Lek watched over the baby, while Saī turned towards Dūan, "One looks to the mother first, unless the baby needs help more." First Saī gave Dūan medicine for the placenta. She rubbed her hands with alum and tried unsuccessfully to work down (*klōm*) the slippery placenta. Then she told Dūan to get on her hands and knees, and exert all the force she could. Dūan crept around the floor but it still did not come. Saī then tried hitting Dūan's back three times with Dūan's own pillow. Finally she gave Dūan a leaf of betel pepper to chew, hoping to induce a wind-producing nausea and so push out the placenta. In the end Dūan resumed her sitting position and it was pressed out. So the baby would not get pimples, the placenta was cleaned carefully, then put into an old pot, mixed with two dishes of salt, and set aside.

While Lek sewed up the partially completed cushion, Saī laid the baby along her legs, and washed him with soap. Sometimes she washed the baby before the cord was cut, if the placenta came quickly. She used salt to remove the greasy fat from his body, though she would have preferred "fermented tamarind to protect him from pustules that enlarge to sores (*rōk phu-phōng*)." "Soft tissue like a stomach covering his head! What a good sign of progress and fortune!" she exclaimed. She powdered him with face powder (*dinsōphōng*), and painted his abdomen with turmeric, "so wind will not make him cry." Covering him with a little piece of old cloth, she laid him on Lek's old winnowing tray (*kradong*).

It was the moment to winnow (*rōn*) the baby, and link it to home and family. While Lek got the holy unspun cord, others placed on the tray with the baby all manner of traditional things to influence the progress and well-being of the child during his lifetime. Saī put on the *phlai*, the clod of soil, and the tapered bamboo she had used to cut the cord "because they will never be used again," but actually these would magically root the child to that house and land. Song laid on a school exercise book and pencil, so that his son would have knowledge and a good memory. Mī got a needle for sharp wit. If the baby had been a girl, the needle would have given sewing skills. When all was in readiness, Dūan had to decide on the ones to raise the child aloft, catch the tray as it was dropped, and bless him as the holy thread was tied on. She had to choose these persons carefully, for the child would later manifest these characteristics. Much as Dūan loved her own mother, Lek ought not to winnow the child because she had had the misfortune to lose three babies in infancy. An older person was desirable, for longevity, too, indicated virtue, and the child would then also live long. Of all the women present, besides her mother, Saī was the one Dūan trusted and respected most, and Saī had raised healthy babies. Dūan turned to her. "Please winnow and bless the baby." She wanted, as every mother did, to catch and so claim the child for herself.

Saī seated herself close to Dūan, picked up and raised high the tray with the little boy and the auspicious items. Waving the tray in a circular motion slowly from left to right, clockwise, she recited the old words: "Three days a spirit child; on the fourth day, a human child! Whose child is this? Is this the child of a female pot? Of a jar? Come, take this child!" Three times Saī chanted these words and on the third, Dūan cried out, "Mine!" The tray with the child was gently tossed in her direction. She caught it as it slid toward her. Then Saī took the holy thread and tied some around each of the child's wrists and ankles to seize and "welcome" its soul (*kānrapkhwan*), giving the while the traditional blessing: "Come *khwan*! Come my own child! Stay well and eat well! Do not get sick or have fever! Be cool and happy! Feed your father and mother until they are old! Hold the walking stick with the gold head, or the stick with jewels on its top! Stay at home like the bottom of the house post! Watch the house like a cat! Eat and stay here! Never go roaming! Be fat as the golden ash pumpkin, heavy as the long melon, strong as an elephant in must! Be the head priest when ordained and the leader of men when you leave the priesthood! Come, *khwan!*"[2] Thus, Dūan claimed the child for herself and for her family, to nourish and raise. Because such a fine person as Saī had started this son on its life-habits, and Dūan was already sparing no efforts in assuring his progress, he would be a good boy, and reciprocate her pain and effort by care in her old age.

The next step was to prepare for Dūan's postpartum days of rest beside the holy fire. Before the baby arrived the fire floor had been prepared, but not lighted. Song had chopped down a banana tree, and quartered and trimmed the trunk into four good planks. Along a wall inside their house he had laid them in a square about three feet on each side and eighteen inches deep. He remembered that at Chaī's birth, the fire had to be in a corner, because of the direction of the celestial Snake. Lek picked up a large round basket and went out to get the soil, which had to come from the north side of the house. Three full baskets she was to get, no less, but there could have been five. She heaped the soil into the frame, smoothing it to a good fire floor. After she poured in the last load, she picked up three handfuls of earth and put them back in the basket. Quickly she took them back to the spot she had been digging and tossed the three handfuls one by one onto the earth, murmuring to the spirit of the land that she was returning the earth she had taken. Back in the house, in each of the four corners of the fireplace, Saī planted a little banana leaf bowl containing rice, sticks of incense, a candle, and flowers. "Some persons add areca nut and betel pepper leaves, but I was not taught to do it that way," she commented. A fire of the *sakāe* wood was laid, and the placenta and cord in the pot placed at the back where they could dry with the heat. To prepare Dūan's bed, Song searched the house for a smooth plank about fourteen to sixteen inches wide. Not one. So he ran over to a neighbor and borrowed a good one! He cut two banana trunk sections to set this plank up so that it was as high as, and two or so hand spans from, the fireplace. Saī checked that firewood, woodpile, and plank were all parallel to the celestial Snake. Then the fire and the incense in the corners were lit.

Meanwhile Saī had been washing the lower part of Dūan's body and legs with warm, boiled water. She painted Dūan's abdomen with tur-

2. Another version added the words, "Have the strength of Hanuman! Hold the stick with the iron head! Be a student!" For a girl, "If you have a family, keep cool and happy! Earn your livelihood (*tham mā hā kin*)! Have enough to use and eat! Do not lower (*tam*) your face, or eyes," i.e., "don't be poorer than your friend." A China-born "Thai" woman's blessing was "Mother, nourish, and care for this child. Do not let it be hurt or have fever."

meric, lime, and alcohol, putting a little on the hands and arms, and now gave her a fresh skirt. "To cure the womb" Saī also gave her a "filtrate" of tamarind, salt, and water to drink, the same potion people also gave to the cherished buffalo on the rare occasions when a calf was born. Finally, she asked Dūan to lie on the floor a moment. Putting her foot on Dūan's hip she pressed hard, three times on each side, to "close the hipbone" and get the pelvis back into place again.

Now that the fire was going nicely and Dūan was "ready to warm her body," the all-important prayer and incantation "to control the hotness and poison" of the fire had to be pronounced lest the mother's body be "swollen or burned." Saī took raw rice, salt, and alcoholic liquor in her mouth, chewed them, and sprayed them over the fire and over Dūan's body three times, saying, "Spirit of the Fire and Wind, may both mother and baby be cool and happy!" and murmuring her secret formula with ancient Pali words about "great fire" and "death." With the shoulder cloth that she always wore to the temple draped diagonally over her left shoulder and under her right arm Dūan knelt and faced the fire. Praying for happiness to the Mothers of the Fire, Fire Floor, and Wind, and finally to the Lord Buddha, the Holy Brotherhood of Priests, and the Sacred Law, she bowed, hands clasped, and touched the floor three times with her forehead. Then she rose and lay down on the plank with the holy fire on her right side.

As Dūan was resting quietly, Saī made three "tapping fruits," balls of tamarind leaves, *phlai,* and salt wrapped in cloth. One was put well up between Dūan's legs to cure the birth wound. The other two were set aside for use on subsequent days. Saī painted the baby's tongue with alcoholic medicine, and from her fingers dropped a little honey and boiled water into his mouth. Then she laid him on his tray on the floor close by Dūan, on the side away from the fire.

—*Jane Richardson Hanks*

48: Birth Customs in the Middle Ages

A picture from an illuminated manuscript—Lydgate's metrical "Life of St. Edmund"—shows the birth of the saint and gives a vivid idea of a medieval nursing chamber. The clothes of the ladies—one of them wears a horned headdress, another a U-shaped one, showing the fretted nets over her ears—their graceful, fitted dresses, as well as the elegant and even luxurious furnishings of the room, show that the scene dates from the later Middle Ages, in fact the fifteenth century, when privacy and comfort were valued more than they were in the early part of the period.

The room is one in which one would not mind sleeping oneself. The mother of the newly born saint sits up in bed, receiving the ministrations of three female attendants, while another one, the lady in the horned headdress, is seated before a blazing log fire. The mother appears to be fully clothed and is wearing a veil, complete with halo, on her head. The head covering is what one would expect, for up till comparatively modern times people were careful to protect their heads from the night air. But it was the usual custom in the Middle Ages to sleep naked in bed. (A woodcut from the *Roman de Mélusine* shows a married couple in bed, wearing nothing but night caps, intently watching a lady who from the text I take to be Mélusine, suckling one of a pair of twins.) Whether some kind of garment was worn during childbirth, I do not know. It seems more likely that the illustrator thought it more decorous to clothe the mother of a saint even in bed.

The bed itself, probably a feather one, is handsome, with a richly patterned canopy and curtains, the sheet neatly folded over a coverlet of the same design. The walls appear to be painted in a floral pattern; the floor is tiled in small squares, and there is a decorative-looking rug in front of the fire, and gold candlesticks, cups, and other vessels in recesses over the fireplace and on top of an open cupboard.

There is an air of indescribable well-being and coziness about the scene, and of that triumphant joyfulness which was summed up once and forever in the words: "but as soon as she is delivered of the child, she remembereth no more the anguish for joy that a man is born into the world."

One of the sculptures on the columns of the Hôtel de Ville in Brussels shows another mother, also belonging to the latter part of the fifteenth century. She wears a turban-like headdress and is seated at the foot of a solid-looking cradle. She has a wistful expression as though she were reflecting more on the cares than on the delights of motherhood, and no wonder, for not only has she a child lying in the cradle, but is suckling a smaller infant who lies naked on her lap. She seems to be meditating on the apparent unfairness of Providence in allotting to women so much the larger share in the production and rearing of children. This theme was the subject of a charming sermon by St. Bernardino da Siena.

St. Bernardino admonished husbands thus: "Wherefore as thou seest that thy wife endureth travail on every side, therefore thou, O husband, if she falls into any need be sure thou help her to bear the pain. If she be with child or in childbirth, aid her in so far as in thee lieth, for it is thy child also. Let all help her whereinsoever they may. Mark her well, how she travaileth in childbirth, travaileth to suckle the child, travaileth to rear it, travaileth in washing and cleaning by day and by night. . . ." He goes on to say: "All this travail seest thou, is of the woman only, and the man goeth singing on his way."

Then comes this engaging anecdote: There was once a baron's lady who said to me, "Methinks the dear Lord our Master doeth as He seeth good, and I am content to say that He doeth well. But the woman beareth the pain of the children in many things, bearing them in her body, bringing them into the world, ruling them, and all this oftentimes with grievous travail. If only God had given some share to man. If only God had given him the child-bearing!"

Did St. Bernardino rebuke the baron's lady for impiety? No, good man that he was, he merely replied, "Methinks there is much reason on thy side."

The everyday miracle is accomplished. The thin, protesting wail of the newborn babe is heard in the birth chamber. The midwife receives the child. Its mouth and gums are rubbed with a finger dipped in honey, its little limbs washed and rubbed with salt and honey, or oil of myrtle and roses before being tightly swaddled in swaddling bands, for it is supposed that without these its limbs will not grow straight. Then it is put in a dark place to sleep for, as a Franciscan monk, Barthélemy l'Anglais, pointed out in a book he wrote about 1350, babies need a great deal of sleep. (He also warned parents to protect the baby's eyes against too strong a light, and against the danger of impure milk.) If it is a child of royal or noble birth it may have a gilded cradle with a fur coverlet.

Now the child must be baptized, for the belief is held that if it dies without baptism, its soul will never reach Heaven, but will be consigned to limbo. What this state of being implied was a questionable point. Some theologians believed that it entailed an eternity of physical torment. Others, like St. Thomas Aquinas, who were unable to accept this atrocious perversion of the teaching of the Saviour who said: "Suffer the little children to come unto me," claimed that the limbo of the unbaptized, though falling far short, of course, of the ineffable bliss of Heaven, was a place of relative happiness. Others again (I think they may well have been parents) cherished the tender belief that these little lost souls were baptized at the feet of Christ. Popular superstition said that they were changed into Gabble or Gabriel hounds, who hunted their despoiler the Devil throughout eternity. When the wind moaned round the house on stormy nights, people told one another that it was the Gabble hounds howling for their prey. It was not surprising that theologians wrote with abhorrence of those priests or midwives who by their negligence robbed the dying infant of its chances of salvation. It may seem astonishing, in the circumstances, that the infant was not usually baptized till the day after its birth, but it must be remembered that in an emergency, and in the absence of a priest, anyone could administer baptism to the dying child: a woman, or even a heretic or a pagan. Medieval theologians held that three circumstances supplemented the actual rite itself—if a child died on its way to church, if it died in the presence of the priest who was about to baptize it, or if it was an abortion born of pious parents who had prayed for its salvation.

Some care had to be exercised in choosing a godmother, for there was a superstition that if a pregnant woman stood as godmother, either her godchild or her own child would die prematurely. (To invite the first poor person met with on the way to church, to act as godfather was thought to bring long life to the baby.) Altogether it was a tricky time. St. Augustine said: "All diseases are to be ascribed to demons, chiefly so they torment the fresh baptized, yea, even the guiltless newborn infant." Women were inclined to rely for protection on obscure and ancient beliefs, forbidden by the Church. There were appropriate spells for each state—prenatal, and before and after the christening.

A woodcut dating from about 1450 shows a baptism. The baby is being held over the font by a woman, while the Bishop holds up his hand in blessing.

The baby's soul having been thus cared for, the next consideration was to keep its body alive. The death rate among young children was cruel throughout the Middle Ages, and for centuries to come, and this is hardly to be wondered at when one considers the elementary state of medical science and of sanitation.

After the breakup of the Roman Empire, the art of medicine fell upon bad times. Surgery, physiology, and medicine itself made hardly any progress, in the earlier part of the Middle Ages at any rate (though the flame of knowledge was kept alight at such centers of medical learning as Salerno and Padua). Disease was generally considered to be a punishment for sin. The Black Death, before whose appalling ravages the physicians were helpless, was popularly ascribed to such diverse causes as Divine Wrath at the introduction of long, pointed shoes, and to the malice of the Jews.

Superstition dictated a number of remedies: "This charme brought Angel Gabriel to Sanctus William for to charm cristen men from worm, from venom, fro goute, fro festyn and fro rankyl." Others were a mixture of exorcism and herbalism: "If a mad hound hath bitten a man, take the seed of flex and stampe it and temper it with holy water and give it him to drink." Others contained fearsome ingredients: "the grease of a rat," "the hair of a dog," "snails that creep in" (i.e., slugs). "A good ointment for the gout. Take an owl . . ." and so on.

There is a masterly simplicity that must be admired about the following: "Give him to drink cristal [ice water?] and if he spew it he shall be dyed."

One wonders how many children who were backward at talking were dosed with this one: "For him that may not speak well give him to drynke houndstongue." Or when they had a toothache underwent this treatment: "Take a candle of mutton fat mingled with seed of sea holly; burn the candle as close as possible to the tooth, holding a basin of cold water beneath it. The worm [which was gnawing the tooth] will fall into the water to escape the heat of the candle."[1]

It is consoling to reflect on the immense number of herbs that were used for medicinal purposes in the Middle Ages. One hopes that quite a number of them may have done good.

The medieval baby's chance of survival might have been even slim-

1. Here, as in the other prescriptions, I have drastically modernized the spelling for the reader's convenience.

mer, if it had not been for the fact that breast-feeding was the accepted custom. In the higher ranks of society, the mother usually delegated this important duty to a wet nurse, and the reluctance of fashionable women to feed their children was fulminated against by both doctors and theologians. There were three reasons, according to one male authority, why these ladies shirked their maternal duties: first because it was not the fashion to give suck, second because they were afraid of losing their figures, and third because they wished to frolic with their husbands (which, the writer added severely, is incontinence).

There were some women of rank however who did their duty in this respect. St. Bernard, who was the son of a noble knight, was first fed with his mother's milk, and afterwards "nourished with greater meats." Then there is the story about the Countess of Boulogne, which not only conveys one in imagination right into the solar or lady's chamber in a medieval castle, but shows the almost mystical significance attached to the act of breast-feeding, and the belief that with the woman's milk the child imbibed something of the woman's characteristics. The close tie that existed between foster mothers and their fosterlings, and between foster brothers, is too well known to need emphasizing.

—*Magdalen King-Hall*

49: Hawaiian Birth Customs

As far back as I can remember, birth was frankly discussed before me. My grandfather, grandmother, and an uncle and aunt were experts in midwifery (*pale keiki*). Grandfather and a granduncle — Kanaka'ole and Keku'ia of Waikapuna, Ka'u[1] — were among those listed by King Kalakaua as noted kahunas (old notebook in Bishop Museum). Grandmother attended herself each time a baby was born to her, until the birth of her last child, when her eldest son helped her. My uncle practiced obstetrics until his death, my aunt until she was too old to work.

My white father, who admired his native mother-in-law, never disapproved of her teachings. But my mother, influenced by her white friends, tried to make me believe the myths commonly told the foreign children. When I was nine years old, I helped my aunt by keeping up the fire to heat water for a confinement. I enthusiastically told a white neighbor that Mrs. D had "borned a new baby," and the following day my mother was visited by a delegation of four white women, who told her that it was not "nice" for me to know of such things. So I helped no more until I entered my teens; then I voluntarily helped my aunt.

I am glad that I learned of the Hawaiian customs and beliefs pertaining to birth and infancy. Often I am asked whether I believe all of the superstitions. What does it matter whether I do or not? These beliefs were part of my people's life.

Prenatal Care

From the fourth moon of pregnancy (*hapai*), diet was regulated. No bitter foods were eaten; no hot things, such as the chili pepper (*nioi'ai*);

---

1. The glottal closure or hamzah is indicated by Bishop Museum by the use of an inverted comma. The hamzah in Hawaiian represents a "k" which has been dropped in the written language but is distinctly heard in Hawaiian speech. In this paper, the hamzah is used in native words (not anglicized in *Webster's New International Dictionary*), proper names, and place names (except the widely-known island names). — Editor.

and no *pupuʻawa* (a shellfish of the genus *Thais*) because of the tartness of the gall. Such foods were believed to affect the eyes of the unborn baby and to leave a bitter taste in the mother's throat when she belched, a condition called *haoa*. Too much salty food was not allowed, and only a little raw fish. The woman was encouraged to eat as much as she could of greens such as *popolo* (*Solanum nigrum*), *luʻau* (young taro leaves, *Colocasia esculenta*), *palula* (young sweet potato leaves), or *ʻaheahea* and mild herb medicines like *koʻokoʻolau* (*Bidens* sp.) and *akiohala* (*Hibiscus youngianus*) blossoms. These and other herbs were eaten "i paʻa ke kino o ke keiki i ka laʻau" (that the herbs build up the body of the child). After the sixth month the pregnant woman was taught to eat lightly, lest she have trouble at birth with a large baby.

The longing for particular foods (called *hoʻokauha*) was considered to be the wish of the child. The obstetrician (*kahuna pale keiki*) read in these longings the nature of the baby. If the mother longed for *manini* fish, it meant that the child would be affectionate, as fond of its home as the *manini* is of its sea pool, and just as shy and timid. If the mother longed for squid, it meant that the child would cling like the squid, but if it did not like a person it would flee (*heʻe*) from him. A desire for *hilu* fish foretold a quiet, industrious child; for tiger shark, a fearless fighter. If the mother vomited constantly during pregnancy, it meant that the child would not be a good provider, for it had shown that it did not care whether the mother had food.

Whatever a parent did during pregnancy affected the nature of the child. If the father and mother were always busy and interested in their work, the baby would be industrious. The mental attitudes of the parents affected the child's disposition. Jealousy of wife or husband was called *ʻiloli*, and was said to be natural during pregnancy.

When a pregnant woman bathed, she was told to move her abdomen to and fro gently (*hoʻoniʻoni*) to loosen the baby so that it would not "stick" at birth.

The kahuna examined his patient at intervals. He passed his hand carefully over the abdomen to see whether the baby was in the right position; if it was not, he oiled his hand with kukui or coconut oil and set to work to manipulate it into the correct position.

If the kahuna wished to discover the sex of the baby, he sat down to talk to his patient, suddenly saying, "Let me see your hand." If the woman extended the right hand, the baby would be a boy, if the left, a girl.

Pregnant women were not allowed to wear leis, lest at birth the umbilical cord strangle the infant (*lei i ka piko*). Stitching tapa or working with cords was not permitted, lest a kink in the cords cause such a kink in the umbilical cord. No pregnant woman was allowed to string fish for drying, for, if a fish should spoil, the baby would have a nose disease that affected the breath. This disease was called the *iʻa-kui* (strung-fish), because during certain months of the year an unpleasant odor, like that of decomposed fish, came from the nose. This disease was incorrectly called *ihu-pilau* (stink-nose).

The changes in the body of the woman were watched as pregnancy developed. A dark line (*alawela*) began to go upward slowly from the bottom of the abdomen and another started down from the top. When these lines met and went into the navel, the baby would soon be born. Nipples that protruded were called *maka-puaʻa* (pig nipples) and those that dented inward a little were called *maka-mino* (dented nipples). My aunt would look at a woman's breast and say, "Ah, *maka-puaʻa*. That is good, easy for the baby to take," or "*Maka-mino*, not so good. Baby's mouth must work before it can hold on." A woman whose breasts flowed from the fourth month of pregnancy was said to have *waiu-koʻa* (always-filled breasts).

Cracking of the skin, caused by scratching, was called *nahaha*. To lessen skin irritation, kukui oil was rubbed on every day. Raw, dry kukui was mashed, wrapped in tapa, and rubbed over the body.

A pregnant woman whose abdomen was very large was said to have a warm bosom (*poli mahana*), which made the baby move forward; a woman who didn't "show" much was said to have a cold bosom (*poli anu*), from which the baby drew toward the spine, where it found warmth.

For two months before the baby was born, the mother ate *ʻilima* blossoms or the thick end of the hau blossoms daily, as the slippery juice was believed to act as a lubricant.

The cry of ʻEweʻewe-iki (Ghost-mother) was said to be the sign that a baby was to be born in the neighborhood. (Not to be confused with the ʻewaʻewaiki, sooty tern.) ʻEweʻewe-iki was a woman who died in childbirth, just as the head of the child appeared. The baby's body remained with her own. Her ghost always flew over the homes of expectant mothers crying, " ʻeweʻewe! ʻeweʻewe!" and the voice of her baby answered, "Nah! nah! nah!" ʻEweʻewe-iki harmed nobody and flew only to tell of a new birth. The only thing that angered the ghost-mother was to hear someone cry out, "Come down here and I'll strangle your baby!" (*Iho mai i ʻumi aku au i ko keiki.*) When ʻEweʻewe-iki was thus angered, she would descend to seek vengeance, but the heat and smoke of a fire would drive her away. I have been told that ʻEweʻewe-iki cried the night

131

before I was born and that Grandmother looked up to the sky and said, "Thank you, we'll look forward to its coming."

Confinement

When the day of birth (*hanua*) arrived, many relatives gathered, some of them to carry out specific duties. Sometimes the woman was seized with a longing to see a certain relative or friend. Such a desire was called *kau ka maka* (setting the eyes on one) and meant that the baby would be very fond of that person. If he could not be present, a member of the family placed a stone before the door, exclaiming loudly, "Here is so and so." This satisfied the patient, as, through the stone she could "feel the presence" of her friend. The stone was later thrown into the sea or some place where it would be safe from pollution. I once threw such a stone into the crotch of an *'ohi'a* tree, where I knew it would be safe as long as the tree stood.

False labor pains were called *ku'ia* and were believed to be sympathetic pains for another childbearing woman in the neighborhood. A woman undergoing sympathetic pains was made to rest and was given warm food to eat until she felt better. However, a competent kahuna knew to the exact hour when the baby was due. He could pass his hand over the abdomen and tell what time of day the child would be born.

Some kahunas knew of a way of giving the labor pains to someone else and letting the mother have a "painless" birth. My uncle and grandfather were said to be experts at transferring pain. The credit was due, I was told, to certain gods worshipped by kahunas. These gods came to their assistance and gave the labor pains to anyone they chose, or to pet animals. I was told of a horse who bore the pains while her mistress gave birth. The last painless birth in our family was when my older sister was born. In the next room slept a lazy relative. My uncle, who was the kahuna, prayed to Haumea (the goddess of birth), and directed that the pain be given to that lazy brother-in-law of his. The poor fellow, who had been enjoying his sleep, began to moan and groan until after my sister was born.

The expectant mother was encouraged to walk to and fro at the beginning of labor, but when the pain became intense, she took a kneeling position with knees apart. A helper sat in the back to act as a support if the patient wished to lean back, or to hold her around the waist. No Hawaiian woman dared scream with pain, lest she make herself the talk of the neighborhood. The kahuna in charge sat in front of the woman. Someone was sent to the beach for the young leaves of the beach morning glory (*pohuehue; Ipomoea pescaprae*) which were supposed to hasten the birth. The number of leaves varied—some kahunas asked for eight, others for sixteen or twenty-four—but were always units of four. The person who gathered the leaves picked half of the desired number with the right hand, addressing a prayer to Ku (the god of medicine), then the other half with the left hand, addressing a prayer to Hina (the goddess of medicine). The two sets of leaves were kept separate, the ones in the right hand to be eaten by the mother, those in the left to be crushed and rubbed over her abdomen. As Ku was the stronger, the leaves eaten were those from the right hand.

Some of my relatives in the country still have faith in the virtue of beach morning glory for childbirth. An old kinswoman told me of a neighbor who had a difficult time in giving birth. She began to swell and turn blue so her husband went for the doctor in a village miles away. As soon as he left, my kinswoman sent the patient's brother for beach morning glory leaves. She rubbed some of the leaves on the patient's abdomen and gave her some to eat. A good brisk *lomilomi* (massage) to the limbs started circulation, and the baby was born long before its father returned with the doctor.

Soon after the amnion (*nalu*) ruptured (*poha*), the baby was born. A reddish-colored amniotic fluid portended a boy, a brownish fluid, a girl. If the baby was large, this fluid would thicken and come away in large clots like thick, dark starch.

A baby that took too long in birth was said to be *kalilolilo* (snatching at life). This worried the kahuna, who resorted to prayers and incantations. A delayed birth might be the result of offending an *'aumakua* (family god). For a member of our family (which numbered several hundred who claimed descent from one of the twin daughters of a gourd that grew out of a dead woman's navel) a gourd was set near or on the head of the patient with a request to the venerable ancestress to come to the assistance of her descendant.

An apparently stillborn baby could be revived by burning the after-birth until it was reduced to ashes. This was done with prayers to Kane-ua-lehu (Kane-of-the-ashes). The heat of the fire was believed to enter the still body in some mysterious way and to animate it. Such a child was considered a kapu child and if it became ill, a little wood ash was always mixed with the herbs with which the child was treated.

The placenta (*'iewe*) was always washed and usually buried under a tree. Failure to wash it caused the baby to have sore, weak eyes. The tree under which the placenta was buried became the property of the child. Some people buried it to one side of a trail or in some other place where it would not be disturbed. In Puna, it was sometimes put on the highest branch within reach on a *hala* tree where the rats would not disturb it. This was said to make the baby's eyelashes stand out prettily like the prickles on a *hala* leaf. People of the other districts sometimes make fun of the Puna folks, calling them *maka kokala* (prickle eyes).

After the mother had borne her child she was given warm broth and herbs to help her overcome the "empty" feeling (*hakahaka*) and expel the excessive blood. Different kahunas had their own choice of herbs and broth. My people liked chicken or fish broth. Tea was made of the dodder vine (*kauna'oa pehu*) or of *ko'oko'olau*. Some put a poi pounder on the abdomen and gently worked it to and fro. If all the blood was not expelled, the mother would have a large abdomen (*'opu-ko'ala*) and look as though she were pregnant all the time. If the placenta was not expelled when it should be, the kahuna pressed with his thumb on the navel of the woman. Her abdomen was bound with tapa after she was washed with warm water, and this binding was done regularly until the discharge ceased.

A bad laceration resulting from childbirth was called *kuka'iku,* a small one *mai* (pronounced mayi). If a woman suffered a laceration, the juice of *ko'oloa* (*Abutilon menziesii*) blossoms or crushed *kukaepua'a* (*Digitaria pruriens*) grass was sometimes used as a healing medicine. Sometimes, warm kukui oil was applied, but if the wound did not heal as it should, the juice of the *pala'a* fern (*Odontoglossum chinensis*) was applied. A woman treated with *kukaepua'a* grass told me that it felt worse than a "chili pepper on the tongue." My aunt preferred warm kukui oil for her patients.

The discharge that came from the womb (*walewale* or *walewale keiki*) continued for about a month. If a woman became pregnant again soon after the cessation of the flow, the second baby was said to be the *walewale* of the first. Conceiving again too soon was ridiculed.

If a woman's menstrual flow ceased for about a year after childbirth, she was said to be *po'o-kapu* (kapu-headed) — "aia a wela ke po'o o ke keiki i ka la" (until the baby's head is heated by the sun). The above saying means until he was old enough to creep or toddle out into the sunlight by himself. This cessation of the menstrual flow for a few months was called *ho'oki'o.*

Care of the Infant
Immediately after a baby was delivered, it was wrapped in a piece of tapa to prevent its taking cold.

The first movements of a baby at birth were always noted. If a child turned to face its mother, it would always love her. (I was told that my first action was to face my mother and grab at her big toe, giving a lusty yell.) If it turned to any relative present, it would love that person best; if it turned its back to its mother and faced the door, it would be fonder of outsiders than of its own people. If born face down it would be fond of chanting, even if it had a poor voice.

The attending kahuna examined the child's body, hands, feet, and head to see if there was anything that needed correction and to foretell what sort of a man or woman it would be.

Arrowroot (*pia*) starch was used back of the ears, under the arms, in the groin, and in any creases of the body, as we use talcum powder today.

The newborn baby was oiled with warm kukui oil. The grandparent in charge sucked the nose of the baby clean after rinsing his own mouth. The removal of the *nalu* or fluid of the nasal passage prevented severe headaches and nasal obstructions (sinus trouble?) later in life. This fluid he spat out, then rinsed out his mouth once more. Asked what the Hawaiians did for sinus trouble, a Hawaiian woman who was well versed in herb remedies answered, "They did nothing, for they never had it. Sinus trouble was killed as soon as a baby was born. Hawaiians of old had good noses."

Next, the grandparent stuck a finger, sometimes wrapped in a clean piece of tapa, into the mouth of the baby, gagging it just enough to disgorge any of the birth fluid that might have slipped into its throat. The eyes were wiped clean and a little of the mother's milk squirted into them.

The umbilical cord was tied with an *olona* (*Touchardia latifolia*) string and cut off with a piece of bamboo, but I saw pen knives used when I was a child. The cord was cut to within about two inches of the navel. To prevent the umbilical cord from being injured, a strip of soft tapa was wound around the child's waist. The baby was not bathed (at least among my people) lest the area around the cord be wet, but a little of the mother's milk was used around the cord. If the cord dropped off too quickly, the baby would feel hungry easily, but, if it took seven or more days for the cord to drop off, the child would be *pa'a ka'opu* (solid in the stomach and able to go a whole day without feeling the pangs of hunger). After the cord dropped off the baby was bathed.

Great care was given the umbilical cord, for if a rat found and ate it, the baby would have the thievish nature of a rat. A thief was called *piko-pau-'iole* (navel-eaten-by-rat). In every district and on every island there were places reserved for disposal of navel cords. Two such places were Ka-papa-a-Hina on Mokuola (Coconut Island, Hilo) and Wailoa, a "stone shaped like a man," in Wailoa stream bed (now filled with dirt).

There was a small hole in the stone just where the navel should be. The cord was pushed into this hole and a pebble shoved after it to cork the hole until the action of the water worked it loose again. In the water close to the shore of Coconut Island is a flat stone, like the top of a table with cracks in it, called Ka-papa-a-Hina. There, the cords were hidden away. *Ola,* the latter half of the name of the island and of the stone, means life and health; so the mothers who wanted life and health for their babies took the cords there. If parents wanted their son to be a navigator and love the sea, the cord was taken out to the ocean and dropped into the sea. Some cords were wrapped in pieces of tapa before being inserted into the holes. A few cords wrapped in human hair were those of beloved children who died before the disposal of the cords. The hair was from the head of a mother, foster mother, grandmother, or any relative who had care of the child. While wrapping the cord, the relative would address the deceased, "O so-and-so, here is a part of my body, my hair. May it be a token of me in the spirit world. Do not come back to hurt us; do not be angry with us. When you wish to come to us, come in love to help us."

The term for a very near relative is *piko* (navel). A person said, "So-and-so is my *piko,*" meaning that he is very closely related to him. To dream of an injury to one's navel foretells death or disaster to a near relative. When the love between relatives had been severed, it was called "moʻ ka piko" or "moku ka piko" (the severing of the umbilical cord). This meant that one would not lend a hand to help his relative, or, if he were to die, mourn him. If the one who injured his brother repented and wished to make peace, he went to a kahuna who knew him and the relative who had disowned him. The kahuna prayed that the severed *piko* be tied once again.

I have seen many old people with small containers for the umbilical cords of the children of the family. These were kept until the opportunity arrived for the proper disposal of them. One grandmother took the cords of her four grandchildren and dropped them into Alenuihaha Channel. When reminded that the two older children were girls, she replied, "They have Oriental blood in their veins too. I have always wished them to be travelers and sail the seas to Japan, to the Philippines, and to Spain from whence their father's ancestors came."

Next to the heiau of Kalae-o-ka-manu at Wailua on Kauai, is Holo-holoku, where the royal babies of old were born. The stone where the cords of these babies were hidden is still there, and in the cracks are the small stones that once held the cords in place.

—*Mary Kawena Pukui*

50: Midwifery

The etymology of her name is of interest. The ancient Jews called her the wise woman, just as she is known in France as the *sage-femme*, and in Germany, the *weise Frau* and also *Hebamme* or mother's adviser, helper, or friend. The English "midwife" is derived from *midwif*, or with-woman.[1] In Spain and Portugal, she is known as *comadre*, while the Latin is *cum-mater*, which is strikingly close to the Spanish and English, and from which it is undoubtedly derived.

There is an old adage that "while midwife and parturient quarrel, the child dies." This, said so pithily, tells eloquently what must have occurred in the lying-in room years ago, and maybe, also, not so very long back. To prove that this assertion is not entirely fiction, I will give some pictures of the English midwife plying her trade a few centuries ago. Dr. Willughby, who practiced as a man-midwife in London, speaks of the "high and lofty conceited midwives, yet will leave nothing unattempted to save their credit and cloak their ignorance." He also tells of a midwife "who, in Threadneedle St., caused several women perforce to hold her patient by the middle whilst that with others pulled the child by the limb one way, and the women her body the other way," yet of another who had her patient tossed in a blanket, "hoping yet this violent motion would force the child out of her body," still of another patient to whom he was called, and whom he "found very pale and faint, having a dying countenance, and her midwife not attending her work, but pulling her by the nose to keep life in her." He also tells of a woman who was so cruelly tortured by the midwife that she determined never to employ one; "and ever since the woman, so soon as she perceived her labor approaching, she causeth a fire to be made in her chamber, and her husband bringeth her into her chamber, and after the taking of their

---

1. J. H. Aveling, *English Midwives, Their History and Prospect.*

leaves one of ye other, he with her desire and consent, locketh her in the room, and cometh no more unto her until she knocketh which is the signe of the delivery to him and such women as are in the house."

Dr. Sermon, quoted by Aveling, says, "some there are (not wanting in ignorance), being over-hasty to busie themselves in matters they know not, destroy poor women, by tearing the membrane with their nails, and so let forth the water to the great danger and hurt not only of the woman, but of the child, which remains dry, the water being sent forth before the time appointed, and sometimes before the child is well turned, which hath been the death of many women and children too."

Now a few words of the manner of midwives: The first English midwife who published a book on midwifery was Mrs. Jane Sharp, London, 1671, entitled *The Midwives Book, or the whole art of midwifery discovered; directing child-bearing women how to behave themselves.*

A few extracts will show some of the peculiarities of her practice:

"The eagle-stone held near the privy parts will draw forth the child as the loadstone does iron, but be sure, so soon as the child and after-burthen are come away, that you hold the stone no longer, for fear of danger."

"It will be profitable, when a woman hath a sore travail, to wrap her back with a sheepskin, newly flead off, and let her lig in it; and to lay a hareskin rub'd over with hare's blood newly prepared, to her belly."

I will now mention an instance of mutilation of children and mothers by ignorant country midwives:

Mrs. Sarah Stone, a midwife of large experiences, "I was sent for to Curry-Mallet, to a tanner's wife, about eleven o'clock at night, it being very bad weather, and bad roads as ever were rode, so that before I got there the child was born. I did not go upstairs directly to see the mother and child . . . when I had dry'd and recovered myself I went upstairs, and to my great surprise saw the child with one eye out, and the whole face much injured, having no skin left on it, and the upper lip tore quite hollow from the jaw-bone, and extremely swell'd, so that the child could make no use of it. . . . I asked the midwife, how the child's face came to be so miserably hurt? She told me the mother fell down two days before she was in travail, and, as she thought, hurt the child, for she was sure she was born right. I told her I was sensible the child came head foremost, but the face presented to the birth; and the damage the child received was from her fingers. She could not make any defense for herself. I found her extremely ignorant."

The practice of midwifery in Great Britain in the eighteenth, as in the previous centuries, was in the hands of women, some apparently highly trained as judged by the standards of the time, but in most cases, in the hands of those utterly devoid of any semblance of training, or even of literacy. From the information available,[2] it seems that these women were under the immediately spiritual jurisdiction of the Church of England, and before the licensure, were obliged to take an oath before the parish minister to whom they were directly responsible for their good behavior and bearing towards their patients. This custom of subscribing to an oath, was, by the by, not peculiar to England, and the other European countries had similar provisions. As the form of oath administered to a midwife about to obtain her license was very quaint, as measured by modern standards, and as it undoubtedly also explained its need for just such contingencies as narrated above, I think it will add to the interest if I recite it *in extenso*:

"You shall swear, first, that you shall be diligent and faithful and ready to help any woman laboring with child as well the poor as the rich, and that in time of necessity you shall not forsake the poor woman to go to the rich.

"Item. You shall neither cause nor suffer any woman to name or put any other father to the child, but only him which is the very true father thereof indeed.

"Item. You shall not suffer any woman to pretend, feign, or surmise herself to be delivered of a child who is not indeed; neither to claim any other woman's child for her own.

"Item. You shall not suffer any woman's child to be murdered, maimed, or otherwise hurt, as much as you may; and so often as you shall perceive any peril or jeopardy either in the woman or in the child; in any such wise as you shall be in doubt what shall chance thereof, you shall thenceforth in due time send for other midwives and other women in that faculty, and use their advice and counsel in that behalf.

"Item. You shall not in anywise use or exercise any manner of witchcraft, charms, or sorcery, invocation or other prayers that may stand with God's laws and the King's.

"Item. You shall not give any counsel or minister any herb, medicine, or potion, or any other thing, to any woman being with child whereby she should destroy or cast out that she goeth withal before her time.

"Item. You shall not enforce any woman being with child by any ungodly ways or means to give you anymore for your pains or labor in bringing her to bed, than would otherwise do.

"Item. You shall not consent, agree, give, or keep counsel that any

2. J.H. Aveling, *English Midwives, Their History and Prospect.*

woman delivered secretly of that which she goeth with, but in the presence of two or three lights ready.

"Item. You shall be secret and not open in any matter appertaining to your office in the presence of any man, unless necessity, or great urgent cause do constrain you so to do.

"Item. If any child be deadborn, you yourself shall see it buried in such secret places as neither hog nor dog nor any other beast may come unto it; and in such sort done as it be not found nor perceived; as much as you may; and that you shall not suffer any such child to be cast into the jaques or any other inconvenient place.

"Item. If you shall know any midwife using or doing anything contrary to any of the permisses, or in any otherwise than be seemly or convenient, you shall forthwith detect, open, or show the same to me or my chancellor for the time being.

"Item. You shall use yourself in honest behavior unto the woman, being lawfully admitted into the room and office of a midwife in all things accordingly.

"Item. That you shall truly present to myself or my chancellor all such women as you shall know from time to time to occupy and exercise the room of a midwife within this aforesaid diocese and jurisdiction of . . ., without any license and admission.

"Item. You shall not make or assign any deputy or deputies to exercise or occupy under you in your absence the office or room of a midwife, but such as you shall perfectly know to be of right honest and discreet behavior, and also apt, able and having sufficient knowledge and experience to exercise the said room and office.

"Item. You shall not be privy or consent that any priest, or other party, shall in your absence, or in your company, or of your knowledge or sufferance baptize any child of any mass, Latin services, or prayers, than such as are appointed by the laws of the Church of England; neither shall you consent that any child, borne by any woman who shall be delivered by you, shall be carried away without being baptized in the parish by the ordinary minister, where the child is born, unless it be in a case of necessity baptized privately according to the Book of Common Prayer; but you shall forthwith, upon understanding thereof, either give knowledge to me the said Bishop, or my Chancellor for the time being.

"All which articles and charge you shall faithfully observe and keep, so help you God, and by the contents of the Book."

— *Morris Braude*

51: Bang Chan Midwives

To deliver a baby as a midwife, or even as an unskilled kinsman, embraced two aspects: a manual or technical, and a magical. These aspects corresponded to Bang Chan's two great worlds of knowledge and experience: the natural and the supernatural.

Midwifery was not alone in embracing both of these categories. Every activity, bus driving, dancing, printing, or other, had its incorporated magical means to augment the probability of success. Though with the manual or technical skills of the natural world alone one could come through all right, with even a modicum of supernatural help, success was greater. No one wanted to take the responsibility and risks of "going it alone," especially when the resources of the supernatural world were so freely and easily accessible to everyone. At the very least, one could start an enterprise on Friday (*Wan Suk*: Happy Day). The closer an enterprise was to the margin of life and death, however, the larger the supernatural element. In farming, curing, and midwifery, for instance, the ritual component was strong.

Since these two worlds were qualitatively different, each required a different method of learning. The supernatural world, immaterial, royal, and sacred, was learned by instruction from a ritually[1] approached teacher. "One cannot accidentally learn. One has to ask to be taught." As a practitioner in this field, the title "*mō*" signalized expertise; where teaching was involved, the title was *khrū* (teacher) or *āčhān* (professor). Speech was the key to this tradition, in spite of sacred books and wall

---

1. To speak ritually one held in the two hands the trio of incense, flowers, and a candle. This was the way to cross over from the profane to the sacred world, to inform (*bōk*) or make a request of, a sacred being (a teacher, priest, king, or deity). The tiny flame of the offering invoked holy fire, and so had the effect of making one's words compelling, for no one could gainsay a request under such circumstances. A husband about to deliver his wife held incense, flower, and candle in hand as he requested the help of ancestors and spirits.

carvings in the temples.[2] Modern education, being book-and-teacher based, shares in this aura. There, even today, listening is more comfortable than reading.

Techniques of the practical, natural world were learned not by teaching but pragmatically by observation, example, and experience. Eyes were the key. "I know because I saw," said a midwife. At the highest level of achievement in the natural world one was expert (*nak*), e.g., convict (*nak thōt*, an expert in being punished) or a tourist (*nak thīeo*, an expert in roaming around).[3] Within the natural world, an intense pragmatism reigned, always emphasizing visual phenomena. People were keenly aware of what they observed and were interested in experimentation. One woman, observing a mother who did not take any medicine, and even ate jackfruit, commented that she was "quite strong." Another watched what happened to a parturient who had no one to boil water for her, so used canal water. "She is healthy!" she exclaimed. Another decided to test whether or not burning up all the wood made a child unable to finish his work and found the maxim untrue.

Just as supernatural knowledge was individually transmitted from a teacher to a pupil, so knowledge learned by observation was personal, even idiosyncratic. The actual observer of a phenomenon might change his ways accordingly, if he wished, but no one else would do so unless he too "saw it with *his* own eyes." The habits of one did not become the habits of another unless the same visual experience had been shared.

Because of the separation of the occult and the practical, the old midwives of Bang Chan would find it inconceivable that technical aspects which are expected to be visually transmitted could be taught from a book.

—*Jane Richardson Hanks*

2. Because words, immaterial and invisible, lay at the base of occultism, words as continuous agents of power, not ony as magical formulae, permeated Bang Chan's ordinary daily life. This was why words, verbal play, and punning might initiate action: pregnant women attended the monks' "coming out of retreat" (*ōk phansā*) so that the child would "come out" (*ōk*) easily.
3. It should not be forgotten that most activities in the supernatural world had their technical sides, and the term "*nak*" was used there too. A curer had to learn his herbs; a dancer, his steps; and a master of ceremonies, the words of the chants.

Polynesia

52: Birth

Slowly the unborn babe distends life's pathway,
   torn by the child's head;
Now the living child,
   long cherished by the mother beneath her heart,
Fills the gateway of life.
There is no room to pass safely through; —
   The child slips downward,
   It becomes visible,
   It bursts forth into the light of day, —
The waters of childbirth flow away.

                —translated by Willard Trask

53: The Ritual of Childbirth

We are Kado, our origin was in Bornu; this is what we do when we have children. It is a little different from the Fulani custom — their women go to their father's compound to have their children.

When you become pregnant you stay in your husband's compound. When you have brought forth your child in your husband's home, and he has been given his name seven days later, on the eighth day they take you to your parents' home. There is feasting and drumming all night, your husband remains hidden. In the morning the grandmother of the child, on the father's or the mother's side, washes the babe and ties him on her back; that is the grandmother who is the midwife. By then the child's mother is able to wash herself, but for the first seven days her cross-cousin came and did it for her, while her mother washed the baby.

But before the child is born, after you have been five months pregnant, you no longer sleep with your husband. You do all the ordinary work until the seventh month, then you do a little less. Round about the seventh month, or earlier, the husband begins to cut down wood in the bush and collect it, he and his younger brother and his joking relations. It they won't help him, his mother will. They collect a large amount of wood. Then at the eighth month the husband's mother buys ginger, potash, cloves, peppers, and all kinds of hot spices. She buys them with her own money. Then she buys honey, and she helps to fetch in the wood. After nine months, one day your husband's mother comes to the door of the hut and calls you. You say, "I'm lying down. I've got a pain in my head." The husband's mother does not come into the hut, she stays at the door and greets you. Then someone from the compound goes to your kinsfolk and tells them that you are lying down. The woman's kinswomen come—her mother's and her father's "sisters," her own "sisters" and her husband's "sisters" and the wives of her husband's elder and younger "brothers." But her own mother doesn't come and her husband's mother stays outside the door of her hut. Her grandmothers come, one is probably her midwife when the child is born, she takes him and cuts the cord and washes him. When he is born the mother covers her head and her eyes so that she shall not see her firstborn child.

If the child is a boy, he drinks only water for the first three days; if it is a girl, for four days. On the third day (for a boy) or the fourth day (for a girl) they take out the uvula and mark him with his family marks. The barber-doctor comes and does it. Then the mother's kinswomen massage her breasts to start the milk flowing, and after the child has had his family marks cut on him, the midwife, the old lady who looks after the baby, brings him to his mother. But the mother refuses to look at him, she refuses to touch him, she hides her hands and covers up her head and face. It is her first child, she is very embarrassed. The father, if it was also his first child, had run away to his friend's compound as soon as his wife's labor began, he stays there hiding. Then the sisters of her father and her mother come and try to make her behave sensibly. But she hides her breasts and her hands, she cries and struggles and pushes away the child. They say "Don't let the child fall, be careful, if the child falls we'll give you a dreadful whipping!" Then they hold her by the shoulders, the midwife holds the baby to its mother's breast, and it sucks the milk. After this they give him water to drink. Then they settle him down on the bed beside his mother—she moves right over to the wall, as far away from her child as she can get. After three or four days comes the naming day. Here in her husband's home the mother won't touch the child, they try to make her but she refuses. The nurse does everything for him. After the naming day they will take the mother to her father's compound, to her mother's hut, and then she will hold her child.

On the day they remove the baby's uvula, the father of the child's father buys a chicken and porridge and stew is made. It is "the day of eating fatness" and everyone eats well. The child's father's mother cooks and makes delicious food for the mother. The midwife grinds up peppers for her, *kimba,* and she eats it. Her husband's mother won't come into the hut until after the naming day. After you have given birth you eat a lot, rich food is made for you with meat, and a great deal of spice and pepper; you eat hot food, you are bathed with very hot water in the morning and evening, there is a fire under your bed—all because you mustn't catch cold. If this is not done you would wither and shrivel up and die with the cold. After seven days of good food and purgatives and washing, you feel strong, you can get up and go outside.

When the seventh day comes round, the naming day, the husband's father kills a ram. The husband's mother brings out a new cloth which she gives to the child's mother, then she ties the baby on the midwife's back and they take him to have his head shaved. In the early morning they give him his name in the entrance-hut, only the *malams* and the men of the family are there. After this the husband's kinsmen distribute three calabashes of kolanuts if the child is a boy, two if it is a girl. The midwife puts him on her back and brings him out to the entrance to be given his name, then she takes him back to his mother's hut. She holds him out to his mother, but she refuses to take him. The sisters of her mother and father come and force her to take him, the mother refuses, they say "You must give him the breast," she will not. At night, her kinswomen come and they fill up the hut. She hides on her bed, and her *kawaye* and younger sisters all sit on the bed and feel the warmth of the fire. When the midwife brings the child and says "Here he is," the *kawaye* and friends of his mother also cover their eyes, they don't want to see the child either. They all rub their teeth with tobacco flowers, they eat kolanuts, they put powder on their faces, they rub their arms and legs with oil, and dress themselves in their best cloths. The mother dresses up too, her friends have stained her arms and legs with henna and done her hair. If anyone says to her "Give the babe the breast," her *kawaye* hide her so that she cannot be seen. But when there is no one about she will take her child and touch him and feed him, there is no one to see. When there are a lot of people there, as there are on the naming day, if the baby cries one of her parent's sisters will lead the mother out of her hut to another one that is empty so that she can suckle the child. The *kawaye* are ashamed of their friend's first child now, but later they will not refuse him anything; your *kawa*'s first child is your own special child. But the child's mother always remains ashamed of him.

After the naming ceremony there is drumming all night, everyone gives away their money; the drummers drum at the entrance of the compound and the womenfolk drum on calabashes in their part of the house. There is no sleeping. When morning comes, at dawn the midwife takes her to the door of her own mother's hut, and she gives the grandmother her grandchild to carry on her back.[1] The mother is washed with hot water, then her mother gives her some gruel, then she gives her her child and she takes him and gives him the breast, she does not avoid him in her own mother's hut, there is no need to. But over there in the compound of her husband it is impossible. Then she eats until she is full and she lies down and goes to sleep. Her mother puts some meat from

1. This custom is called *bangwalle* or returning home. There are many variations as to the time at which the mother returns to her parents' home, how long she stays, etc., and in some cases she may not go at all.

the ram of the naming feast into the stew, she gives her porridge and hot spices, the mother must eat good food.

Then the midwife returns to her own home, her work is finished. She is escorted to her home with her gifts, other older women of the family escort her. She receives the head of the ram, its skin, some of its internal organs, salt, locust-bean cakes, guineacorn, peppers, spices, potash, and powdered spices. She takes all the child's mother's spinning things, she takes them away with her — the mother must not spin for forty days. After that her own mother will buy her some more things for spinning.

On the day that they cut out the child's uvula they give him his family marks. If it is a girl they also cut a little bit off her clitoris, a very little. When our forefathers came south from Bornu they gave up the Barebare marks that you sometimes see, the very heavy ones all over the face; the barber-doctors here can't make them. We adopted the long straight line down the forehead and nose with two little ones here under the eyes — you see the one on my nose is still there, but the others have died out. When the clitoris is clipped the little bit is put on the lintel over the door of the mother's hut. When the child is born the afterbirth is washed and put in a big fragment of a broken cooking pot; then it is buried behind the hut with the cord. When the rest of the cord dries and falls off it is also buried behind the hut, but not in a pot. All this is the midwife's work. The barber-doctor is given spices, the ribs and liver of the ram, salt, locust-bean cakes, peppers, ginger, potash, ten kolanuts, a calabash of corn, and three thousand cowries. Nowadays they give him three or four shillings instead of the cowries. Some fathers refuse to have the child's uvula cut out, then the barber-doctor gives the mother some medicine to cook and give to the baby, so that the uvula shall burst and heal and no longer be there. If they don't cut it and they don't give him the medicine to drink, they may hang a piece of the root of pawpaw round his neck to heal the uvula. Sometimes if the child is a girl, the father also refuses to allow the clitoris to be cut. But the mother will never refuse to have this done, she wants her daughter to grow big and strong. If you do not clip the clitoris you will see the girl getting ill, she gets thin until she dies. If she starts to become like that, and the clitoris is clipped, and medicine put on, then she recovers.

At present I am midwife to four women, they are all pregnant, and in the coming rainy season they will be delivered. I will take the child and put him on my back and carry him about, I will wash him and make him very nice. I will be given the naming day food to eat. There is my younger brother's wife, his mother was my father's sister, so he is my cross-cousin. There is Gude, her husband is my younger brother, he and I are the children of two brothers. There is Almajara, her husband is also my younger brother, he and I are the children of brothers; and it is the same with 'Yardada. You see, if your father's elder brother has children, they are your brothers and sisters, but slightly different from your own brothers and sisters. But you call them "elder brother" and "younger brother" according to whether they are older or younger than you are; if they are younger they are your younger brothers, even though their father was your father's elder brother. Settled Fulani are different, they would call all the children of their father's elder brother "elder brother," whether the children are really older or younger than themselves. We are Habe, we are different. Then too, Fulani won't let their children be adopted, they don't like their laughter taken away to another compound; the child is their laughter and pleasure. We give children to our kinsmen, if they have none of their own we cannot refuse them.

If the child is your first, you remain in your mother's hut for six months, you lie on the bed over the fire, your mother washes you with hot water morning and evening for forty days. On the fortieth day after the birth, alms are distributed to the nearby compounds; porridge is made and a food made from millet-flour and sugar, and about this time (9:30 a.m.) alms are taken to the compounds round about and everyone says "Are the forty days over? Allah be praised! May Allah preserve the child!" The food is taken to the compounds of the kinsfolk, and everyone is given a little; the children take it round. There is no drumming or dancing, only the distribution of the food. About five or six *mudu* of grain would be used for the porridge; people with a lot of grain might use ten. The child's mother adorns herself, the baby is dressed up and one of the little girls ties him on her back and takes him round the compounds of all his kinsfolk. Everyone takes up the child and plays with him and sings to him like this:

> *Child here, I don't want to hear you crying,*
> *When you cry, my mind is upset,*
> *My heart is broken.*
> *Child here, I don't like to hear you crying.*
> *Mother too, she doesn't like to hear you crying,*
> *Father's sister too, she doesn't like to hear you crying,*
> *Mother's sister too, she doesn't like to hear you crying...*

We sing the song for all the kinswomen. Then we sing to him:

> *This child is the father's sister's child,*
> *This child is the mother's sister's child,*
> *You are* goggo's *child,*
> *You are* inna's *child,*
>   *You are children of Habe people.*

If a settled Fulani has married a Kado, then we mix up Fulani and Hausa and sing the song with the Fulani names for the Fulani kinswomen and the Hausa ones for the Hausa. You know we're Kado, Habe, we Bare-bare, people of the country; we didn't come from another country like the Fulani.

Then when the baby cries the little girl who brought him picks him up and ties him on her back and takes him home to suck. It is on the fortieth day that she takes him to the compound of his father's kin, the next day she takes him to his mother's kin. If the little girl gets tired of sitting there while they play with him, she runs off home, and if the baby cries one of the kinswomen puts him on her back and takes him home to his mother. They collect about two thousand cowries for him and take him back with his money. Next day he goes to his mother's kin to be seen, they sing to him and play with him and send him home with two thousand cowries.

The child's grandmother, his mother's mother, is his foster mother, she washes him and carries him about on her back. When she is tired his grandfather takes him and plays with him, he says "Hallo ugly one — Oh but you're ugly!" or "You with the great big head, the huge head!" Your grandparents give you your nickname and sometimes everyone calls you by it all your life, you can't stop them.

After forty days the mother only washes in the morning; altogether she goes on washing for five months. When the sixth month comes, or the seventh, the mother's kinsfolk collect presents for her as they did for her dowry. They get two sacks of rice and two of guineacorn — one from her father's and one from her mother's kin; salt and locust-bean cakes and ten or twenty bottles of oil, groundnut oil or palm oil or butter. Five cloths are given to her by her mother's side and five by her father's side. Except for the two cloths they gave her on the child's naming day, her husband's family don't have to give the mother anything. In the hus-band's compound they cook porridge and stew, millet paste, and chick-ens, they buy sour milk; when the mother's kinsfolk have eaten the midday meal they collect together her "dowry," some other woman ties the baby on her back and the mother covers her face and head and goes along with her kinswomen. The drummers go with them all the way to the husband's compound. The settled Fulani make a procession round the market to show everyone the "dowry," but we go straight to the husband's home. When they arrive the praise-singers call out "Here is the daughter of so-and-so, the grand-daughter of so-and-so, see she has returned home safely!" The drummers and praise-singers are given money. Her hut has been swept out and when she comes in the mother goes straight to her hut. The child has returned to his father's house. The mother will no longer refuse him the breast when her husband's kins-women bring him. But even when he is grown up his parents will not talk to him if there is anyone there, only if they are alone privately with him. They never use his name, they address him "You, son," "You, daughter," or "That son," "Son there." When he is old enough to understand he learns that his parents are ashamed of him. With the second child there is some shame, but after that there is none with the others. But you never look directly at your first child. No one must be able to say "They pick up their first child, they fondle him, they have no shame, they look straight at their eldest child!" If the mother is alone with him she picks him up, she fondles him, she talks to him.

There are other relatives whose names we never use: the husband's "mothers" are called "Mother of . . ." one of their other children. You must not utter your husband's name, either. Your husband's father is "Maigida" — "Master of the house" — unless the marriage is between kin, when he is already your father, so you go on calling him "Baba," "Father." Your husband's elder brothers and their wives you call "Yaya," his elder sister and her husband are "Yaya" too, like your own elder brothers and sisters. But you joke with his younger brother and you joke with all your husband's joking relations — his grandparents and cross-cousins. Your husband's mother will say "Daughter there, do so-and-so," you will reply "Yes, Mother of Mairo," or "Yes, Mother of Abubakar." If she has no other child besides your husband, so there is no other name you can use, you may say "Mother." You may sit and talk with her. My first husband's mother, Duma's mother, was my father's sister, so I just kept on calling her "Goggo," "father's sister." You don't chat with your husband's father, you just kneel down and greet him.

Two years after the child's birth, one of the child's grandmothers, usually his father's mother who often lives in the same compound, comes at dawn and knocks on the mother's hut door; she goes in and picks up the child and takes him or her off to her own hut. The child's mother runs off to her own mother's home. In the morning the child bursts out crying, he cries bitterly. Then his grandfather, the father of his father, writes a text on his board and washes off the ink and gives the child the ink of the text to drink,[2] then the womenfolk make gruel and he

2. Drinking the ink used in writing Koranic texts on a writing board is one of the standard techniques of Hausa protective magic and piety, and is usually performed at least once a day by pious adults during the annual feast of Ramadan. It is intended to ensure that the child grows strong and healthy after weaning. He has, of course, been eating solid food for a long time before weaning, in addition to his mother's milk.

drinks it. He keeps running to his mother's hut, but he doesn't see her there and he bursts out crying. After three or four days he forgets about the breast. His grandmother has him in her hut and she looks after him. After fourteen days the mother's kinsfolk collect "dowry" for her at their compound, basketfuls of rice, millet, guineacorn, salt, bean cakes, locust-bean cakes, and her kinswomen bring her to her husband's home. When she arrives everyone says "Allah give us the bird on the back!" "Allah give us all the health!" Everyone comes to rejoice, the mother dips in to the food they have brought and gives everyone a little, both the people of the compound and any visitors who may come. When her child sees her he rushes to her and she pushes him away and says "Go on, run off to your own hut!" His grandmother picks him up and comforts him, then he comes back to his mother, and the grandmother carries him off to her own hut. Here is the father's mother's hut, here is the child's mother's hut, quite close to one another. Some children put up with it and stay in their grandmother's hut, some don't and come back to their mother's hut and stay there. Sometimes the child is adopted into another compound, a father's sister or a mother's sister, or one of the grandparents, adopt him. The child's own parents give him to her and she carries him on her back. The kinsfolk of the child's father usually take the first child, and the kinsfolk of the mother take the second. Sometimes the third child is also adopted, but the rest usually stay in their mother's hut. It is we Habe who do that, we give our child as a gift to someone to carry on their back. Fulani won't give their child to a brother, they don't want their laughter taken to another compound. They laugh and are happy with the child, they won't let him go to another house. If they marry a Habe woman perhaps they will give away a child, but they wouldn't do so on their own. Even if the mother dies, they leave the children in her hut and the father looks after them.

Before a wife has borne a child her own kin send her gifts at the two annual feasts — rice, guineacorn, salt, locust-bean cakes — at every feast they send her these gifts.[3] When she has a child they give her all the "dowry" for a birth, and after that they make no more gifts to her at the feasts. As I never had a child, my parents always sent me things every feast — sweetmeats, guineacorn, rice, salt, locust-bean cakes, my father

3. These gifts link the two *rites de passage* — a woman's first marriage, and her first childbirth with its *bangwalle* or returning home ritual. Parenthood is the fulfillment of marriage to the Hausa, but under a system permitting polygamous marriage, the husband may already be a parent by another wife, and it is therefore appropriate that the woman's kinsfolk should carry out the exchanges which center about the daughter during the period of her first marriage and first childbirth, and serve as effective links between the two rituals.

and my parents sent them, even after Father had moved to Giwa. My husband rested from taking grain out of his granary, he bought no salt or things for stew, the food they sent would last us for about twenty days. Your family does that because you have not brought forth your child, and yet they want you to feel happy and stay in your hut, and not get up and leave your husband. You see, the husband has paid them a great deal of money, so the wife's family keep on returning the gifts until there is a child. The husband rests from providing food. They don't want their daughter to see her hut bare and go off on her own; if she has a child she will not want to go away.

If a lot of children have died and then one lives, they take her and lay her down at a place where paths meet, near the compound. Whoever comes along and sees the baby on the road says "Look, there's my slave—lost property!" Then he would bring a leather lead like they used to use for slaves when they traveled about, and a ring, he would tie the lead around her neck with a ring in front and one behind, and it wouldn't be removed until she married. They put on the lead, she was a "slave who had been found," but she stayed in her father's compound. She would be called "Ba'i" and the man who had found her always called her "Slave." When it was time to marry her, her "master" would come and claim his ransom money. One would ask for five shillings, one would ask for ten shillings. The father's and mother's kin collected the money and ransomed their daughter. It was just the same for the boys, they were called "Bawa."

Mother's Milk

We call mother's milk the "child's judge"—it always silences him; if he cries, give him the breast, he sucks and is satisfied and then he is quiet! When a child is seven days old we rub the soles of his feet with his mother's milk to kill the flesh there, then even in the dry season he won't feel the heat of the path. If the mother's milk gets onto the child's genitals it will kill them too; you know Sankira, the man who sweeps up the market here in Giwa, he also dances and is a praise-singer—he's not well. The thing that causes a person to be ill in this way is that his mother has not been careful when she is suckling him; she should always cover her other breast with her cloth, so that no milk shall fall on her child's genitals. If milk falls on them they will die. If the child is a boy he won't be able to do anything with women; if a girl, there will be no entrance, it will be blocked up, or her genitals will die. Her husband will send her away, she won't be able to bear children. If it is a man he will not seek after women. Some of these people are hard-working, they make money and put it by. Some of them work very hard at farming, we had one in our *rinji* at Karo, he worked very hard indeed, but he did not go after women, he had no power. He was one of our slaves and he worked a lot, he was very hard-working. Then there was a girl who was not healthy, she came here to New Giwa, she came from the south; her name was Shekara. She was beautiful with light reddish skin. She said she wished to be a *jakadiya*—to Fagaci. He desired her, she was very beautiful with her firm round breasts, but after a short time she left his compound. The children kept on singing at her,

> *She's blocked up, she's only looked at,*
> *Without a door, without a path*[4]

It was a pitiful thing. They kept on and on, we told them "For shame, to behave so unkindly to her!" At first it was said to be a lie, but indeed it was true. Closed up, who would touch her? She stayed here for about six months, she was Fagaci's *jakadiya* but since there was no entrance he sent her away. She used to come to our house to grind grain for us, the children were plaguing her. I drove them away, I said, "If Allah has willed this on her, will you also ridicule her like that?" She said "Indeed, you are right." She came and ground grain in our house, later she went away but I don't know where she went. A lovely girl. There was Danzuma, too, when he was circumcised it putrefied and fell off, then they gave him medicine and it healed. But he was not able to do anything with women.

A mother should not go to her husband while she has a child she is suckling. If she does, the child gets thin, he dries up, he won't get strong, he won't be healthy. If she goes after a year, the child won't get strong; but if she goes after two years it is nothing, he is already strong before that, it does not matter if she conceives again after two years. If she only sleeps with her husband and does not become pregnant, it will not hurt her child, it will not spoil her milk. But if another child enters in, her milk will make the first one ill. If she must go to her husband, she should take a kolanut and sew it up in leather into a charm and wear it round her waist; when she weans her child that is that, she throws away the charm and does as she wishes, then there is another child. It is not sleeping with the husband that spoils her milk, it is the pregnancy that does that. But if her husband desires her, then in the day she carries her child, at night she carries her husband—this is what pleases Allah. He does not like argumentative women. But it is not right that she should

4. Songs of ridicule are generally leveled at sexual offenses, such as premarital pregnancy and incest, and at inability to perform intercourse.

sleep with her husband for two years; if he insists she should wear the kolanut charm. As you know, there is medicine to make the pregnancy "go to sleep," but that is not a good thing.

There was my granddaughter Dantambai, her mother was the granddaughter of my father Malam Buhari; Dantambai was Musa's head wife. When she came to wash, after she had given birth to a child, her mother who bore her came to wash her at her husband's compound. Her mother slept in the hut with Dantambai and the baby. Before five months had elapsed her husband desired her, he crept up to the hut when her mother was asleep and beckoned to her — like this. She got up and went out to him, she also wanted him. Her mother woke up while she was away with him. In the morning her husband came to the hut to greet his mother-in-law. Dantambai's mother was angry, she scolded him, she said "What is the reason for this work? You have three other wives." He was silent. Again he came, she slipped out, and they did as they pleased. Her mother was very angry and said she would return to her own home. When people asked her why, she said it was nothing. But her kinswomen said "Ap. She is going to her husband's hut!" She was spreading scandal. Dantambai's husband had his sleeping hut in the middle and the huts of his four wives round it; it was quite easy to go from her hut to his. Her husband Musa was the son of my *kawa* Kande; Dantambai was my granddaughter. Her mother went to Musa's mother Kande, and told her she was going home. She told her the reason. Kande said "At five months one goes to the husband's hut?[5] Doesn't she want the child to be healthy?" She sent for Musa, her eldest child, she said "Of the South Gate, have you no shame?" She lectured him.[6]

Dantambai became pregnant eight months after the first child was born; for seven months he drank milk, then he drank "pregnant milk" until when she was near to her time they weaned him. When Dantambai knew she was pregnant they sent for her mother, but she was angry and said she would not come. Dantambai and her husband were delighted, but their parents were angry. They said they would give her medicine so that the pregnancy should lie down but he refused, he said "Here is one child, let's have the other one too!" If you go back to your husband's hut, what do you expect? The second child was born after a year, there was already a child on her back, then there was the infant, they were both

5. The point of this tale is that intercourse occurred during the period of the postnatal ablutions.
6. "Of the South Gate" — i.e., "One born at the South Gate," name avoidance between a woman and her eldest child. It is an index of the gravity of Musa's behavior that his mother should speak to him about it directly instead of getting another relative to do so.

being suckled. They sent for me and I said the elder child must be taken to the market in the very early morning, and when the butchers killed a bull they must get the stomach of the bull while it was still warm and rub the child's whole body with it, then the woman who took him must tie him on her back and bring him back to the compound at once. Then she must wash him all over with warm water, and get some butter and rub him with it. Every market day at Zarewa for two weeks, that is seven market days, they did this. Then he was all right; he ate food — gruel and *tuwo* and *fura* and sour milk, he was weaned after a year. He grew strong and well, the children are both alive and healthy now. The new pregnancy spoils the milk and the child ails. But when his body was rubbed with the bull's stomach, then he passed a lot of urine, then his body became strong.[7] These two brothers are young men now, they have both been married recently. She went back to her husband because he desired her very much and she desired him; she was his head wife, he had three others, but she was the one he preferred.

—Baba of Karo

7. Presumably Baba's treatment was intended to cause the child to pass all the "pregnant milk" out of his system. The bull is symbolic of strength and sexual vigor.

54: On the Birth and Rearing
of Children (from the "Sho-Rei Hikki")

In the fifth month of a woman's pregnancy, a very lucky day is selected for the ceremony of putting on a girdle, which is of white and red silk, folded, and eight feet in length. The husband produces it from the left sleeve of his dress; and the wife receives it in the right sleeve of her dress, and girds it on for the first time. This ceremony is only performed once. When the child is born, the white part of the girdle is dyed sky blue, with a peculiar mark on it, and is made into clothes for the child. These, however, are not the first clothes which it wears. The dyer is presented with wine and condiments when the girdle is entrusted to him. It is also customary to beg some matron, who has herself had an easy confinement, for the girdle which she wore during her pregnancy; and this lady is called the girdle-mother. The borrowed girdle is tied on with that given by the husband, and the girdle-mother at this time gives and receives a present.

The furniture of the lying-in chamber is as follows: Two tubs for placing under-petticoats in; two tubs to hold the placenta; a piece of furniture like an armchair, without legs, for the mother to lean against;[1] a stool, which is used by the lady who embraces the loins of the woman in labor to support her, and which is afterwards used by the midwife in washing the child; several pillows of various sizes that the woman in childbed may ease her head at her pleasure; new buckets, basins, and ladles of various sizes. Twenty-four baby-robes, twelve of silk and twelve of cotton, must be prepared; the hems must be dyed saffron color. There must be an apron for the midwife, if the infant is of high rank, in order that, when she washes it, she may not place it immediately on her own knees: this apron should be made of a kerchief of cotton. When the child

1. Women in Japan are delivered in a kneeling position, and after the birth of the child they remain night and day in a squatting position, leaning back against a support, for twenty-one days, after which they are allowed to recline. Up to that time the recumbent position is supposed to produce a dangerous rush of blood to the head.

is taken out of the warm water, its body must be dried with a kerchief of fine cotton, unhemmed.

On the seventy-fifth or hundred and twentieth day after its birth, the baby leaves off its baby linen; and this day is kept as a holiday. Although it is the practice generally to dress up children in various kinds of silk, this is very wrong, as the two principles of life being thereby injured, the child contracts disease; and on this account the ancients strictly forbade the practice. In modern times the child is dressed up in beautiful clothes; but to put a cap on its head, thinking to make much of it, when, on the contrary, it is hurtful to the child, should be avoided. It would be an excellent thing if rich people, out of care for the health of their children, would put a stop to a practice to which fashion clings.

On the hundred and twentieth day after their birth, children, whether male or female, are weaned.[2] This day is fixed, and there is no need to choose a lucky day. if the child be a boy, it is fed by a gentleman of the family; if a girl, by a lady. The ceremony is as follows: The child is brought out and given to the weaning father or sponsor. He takes it on his left knee. A small table is prepared. The sponsor who is to feed the child, taking some rice which has been offered to the gods, places it on the corner of the little table which is by him; he dips his chopsticks thrice in this rice, and very quietly places them in the mouth of the child, pretending to give it some of the juice of the rice. Five cakes of rice meal are also placed on the left side of the little table, and with these he again pretends to feed the child three times. When this ceremony is over, the child is handed back to its guardian, and three wine cups are produced on a tray. The sponsor drinks three cups, and presents the cup to the child. When the child has been made to pretend to drink two cups, it receives a present from its sponsor, after which the child is supposed to drink a third time. Dried fish is then brought in, and the baby, having drunk thrice, passes the cup to its sponsor who drinks thrice. More fish of a different kind is brought in. The drinking is repeated, and the weaning father receives a present from the child. The guardian, according to rules of propriety, should be near the child. A feast should be prepared, according to the means of the family. If the child be a girl, a weaning mother performs this ceremony, and suitable presents must be offered on either side. The wine drinking is gone through as above.

—Lord Redesdale

2. This is only a nominal weaning. Japanese children are not really weaned until far later than is ordinary in Europe; and it is by no means uncommon to see a mother in the poorer classes suckling a hulking child of from five to seven years old. One reason given for this practice is, that by this means the danger of having to provide for large families is lessened.

55: A Zuñi Childbirth

A typical labor case observed by the writer occurred at midnight, October 20, 1896. A child wife, not more than fifteen years old, gave evidence of approaching parturition. She suffered from that time until six o'clock in the following evening, when she was delivered. Owing to the absence of her mother in Ojo Caliente, a farming district, the girl was confined in her mother-in-law's house. She wore only the camis, which leaves the arms exposed, and was covered with a heavy blanket. She lay most of the night on sheepskins spread on the floor near the south end of the room, pressing her feet during the pain against the ledge at the south wall of the room. She changed positions from her side to her back and often lay face downward. The mother-in-law, who was a doctress, had no professional part in the treatment of her daughter-in-law, but took a seat on the floor beside the girl, offering no assistance. The two grandmothers of the girl were present and were much concerned over her suffering. The father, the father-in-law, and a paternal uncle were in an interior room. Their faces expressed anxiety, and they spoke in whispers. The husband of the girl, not expecting the birth of the child for several days, was absent at his farm in Ojo Caliente. The pains increased, and at four o'clock in the afternoon, two doctresses having been summoned, the kneading of the abdomen began. Each doctress took her turn, bestowing much strength and energy on the manipulation. With each pain the girl turned on her right side and caught the belt of the doctress before her, while the second doctress pressed hard upon the back, the girl pressing her feet against the ledge. The labor being prolonged, a doctress held the nostrils of the patient and blew into her mouth, occasionally releasing the pressure upon her nose for an instant. This heroic treatment appears cruel in the extreme, but it is supposed to force the child into the world. The girl wept continually. The sympathy expressed by the relatives and doctresses was enough to unnerve the sufferer. The juniper tea was frequently drunk and the girl occasionally stood over the urinal during the day, but did not leave her bed after four o'clock. Rupture of the membranes occurred an hour and a half before the birth of the child. Half an hour previous to delivery, one of the doctresses made an examination by inserting her hand. Apparently discouraged and alarmed, she notified the mother-in-law of her intention to call upon the officers of the Great Fire fraternity to come and sing their songs. This fraternity has four songs addressed to the Beast Gods for hastening delayed delivery. Should the child be born after the first song, the singing ceases, and so on. Should the child not be born soon after the fourth song, the heart of the patient is bad; the songs are not repeated, and the theurgists leave the house. Accordingly, the mother-in-law provided the doctress with a quarter of mutton and many yards of cotton and calico as an advance payment to the theurgists. For a long time the doctress was unsuccessful in her efforts to find the men, but she persisted in her search and finally returned with them just as the girl was being delivered of a male child. The four theurgists departed at once with the medicine of the Beast Gods and their rattles. As soon as the child's head was exposed, the girl was at once turned upon her back and most vigorously kneaded. Her drawn knees were held by two women and a doctress took her seat upon the ledge between the girl's knees and pressing her hands to the sides of the infant's head, assisted the birth by slightly shaking the child as she pulled it to her.[1] Another doctress severed the umbilical cord with a steel knife, while the doctress holding the child pressed the cord close by the umbilicus until a cotton cord as thick as a lead pencil was procured and wrapped around it several times. In the meantime the abdomen of the young mother was manipulated until the placenta passed. It was held by the umbilical cord and hastily taken from under the blanket on the left side, dropped into a bowl, and carried from the house by the girl's maternal grandmother, who deposited it in the river with a prayer that the young mother might be blessed with many children. While this was happening the mother bit upon a white pebble, that the child's teeth might be strong and white. There seemed to be no evidence of life in the child for an hour after birth, still the doctresses and the paternal grandmother of the girl never ceased their efforts to produce respiration by pressing the nostrils, blowing into the mouth, manipulating the chest, and moving the arms, held outward above the head. Warm cloths were kept around the body and over the

1. Though it is the aim of each doctress present at childbirth to bring the child into the world in order that if it be a boy, he will enter the ki'witsine of her husband, there is no evidence of unfairness toward one another.

head. There was great rejoicing when the faintest sign of life was discovered, but it was fully another hour before respiration was such as to give real hope of life for the child. The writer was surprised at the success of these patient efforts, as the case seemed to be a hopeless one. When no further anxiety was felt for the little one, the doctress called for piñon gum which had been boiled and, chewing it until it was white and pliable, mixed mutton grease with it, and then the paternal grandmother of the girl rubbed it on the stone floor until she produced a roll one-half inch in diameter and about four inches long. A blanket was now folded over the upturned feet and the extended legs of the doctress, who laid the child upon the blanket, its head resting against her feet. Opening the wrappings about the child, she raised the umbilical cord, which was about two and one-half inches long and heavily wrapped with the cotton cord previously referred to, and encircled the umbilicus with the roll of piñon gum; then fluffing some carded wool and making an opening in the center, she drew the wrapped umbilical cord through, patting the wool over the piñon gum. This dressing, which was very clumsy, protruded more than an inch. The abdomen was covered with a bit of solid cotton cloth, laid on warm, and the child's head was kept covered with a warm cloth. The paternal grandmother of the infant now dropped water upon its scrotum, and the doctress rubbed it over the parts, manipulating the penis until its form could be seen. The child's nose was frequently pinched, and the mouth and eyes were delicately manipulated. The latter when closed resembled the eyes of a frog, the lids protruding to a remarkable degree. The child's arms were now placed by its side and it was wrapped in a piece of cotton cloth and a tiny blanket, and these were held in place by strings of yucca over the shoulders, breast, and lower portion of the legs. The child was then laid upon· a folded blanket. Meantime the young mother stood unassisted over the urinal, wrapped her belt around her to hold in place a heated stone, and took her seat on the ledge. Two women removed the sheepskin on which was a pool of the lochial discharge; this the maternal grandmother covered with sand, and the sand was then swept into a cloth and carried out. The girl then drank a cup of commercial tea without sugar,[2] which she enjoyed. After the young mother had taken this nourishment the father-in-law and mother-in-law brought a quantity of damp sand and deposited it upon the floor. One of the doctresses divided the sand into two portions, placed a hot stone slab under one portion and another slab on top of the sand, and worked the sand about the stones until it was thoroughly dry

2. There is great prejudice against the use of sugar at such times. The Zuñi doctors forbid the sweetening of tea or coffee.

and heated, when she removed the stones and placed them with the other part of the sand, which was heated in the same manner. The second portion of sand was made into a circular mound, in which an elliptic depression was formed and made perfectly smooth. A circular depression to fit the child's head was made west of the ellipse, and a ridge of sand was raised between the two depressions to support the child's neck. Over the sand a heated cloth was laid. At this time much disappointment was felt that neither of the ears of corn which were brought by the mother-in-law was a ya'pota (perfect ear). One ear had three plumules, symbolizing fecundity; the other was a single ear. The latter[3] was held, pointing upward, back of the child's head by the mother-in-law, who also held the child. A basket of prayer meal was deposited at the head of the sand bed by the doctress who received the child into the world, and the latter offered a long prayer to A'wonawil'ona for long life and health to the child.[4] After the prayer the doctress raised the cotton cloth and sprinkled a line of meal from east to west over the sand bed, symbolic of the straight path the child must follow in order to receive the blessings of A'wonawil'ona and the Sun Father. The cloth was then returned to its place, the child was laid upon the bed, and the single ear of corn was placed at its left side. The maternal grandmother covered the child with a small blanket, which was a gift from herself. The doctress then struck the sides and ends in turn of a quaint little stool against the floor at the head of the bed, with the seat next to the bed. An Apache basket tray was inverted over the child's head, one side resting on the edge of the stool, the other on the blanket covering, so as to raise from the face a cotton cloth which was thrown over the head. A small blanket was placed over the cotton covering. An occasional faint sound was to be heard from the infant, which caused genuine delight to the family and friends. The mother-in-law next proceeded to prepare the mother's bed with the second portion of sand, first heating the sand in the manner described. The ear of corn having three plumules was placed to the left of the bed, and when the young mother took her seat upon the bed, a bowl of mutton stew, a basket of mush boiled in corn husks, and a basket tray of wafer bread were deposited on the floor beside her. A number joined in the meal, none eating with more relish than the young mother, who sat up an hour and a half. During the meal the paternal grandfather of the infant came from the inner room. At this

3. For a boy the single ear of corn, called the father, is used; a divided one, called the mother, is placed by a girl.
4. The Zuñis believe that the span of life is marked out at birth. This belief, however, does not prevent their incessant prayers to A'wonawil'ona (the supreme power) for health and a long life.

moment the child gave its first vigorous cry, which delighted all present, especially the grandfather. One hour after the birth of the child the mother's pulse was eighty. At the first peep of the sun on the morning following the birth, the doctress who delivered the young mother, having been supplied with a vase of warm water, a gourd, and a basket of ashes, proceeded to bathe the infant. Dipping a gourd of water, she filled her mouth, and pouring the water from her mouth over the head of the child, washed its face and head, rubbing quite vigorously, after which ashes were rubbed over the face, a quantity adhering to the skin.[5] The infant's paternal grandmother now folded a blanket and laid it over the extended legs of the doctress, who placed the infant upon the blanket, its head against her upturned feet. The doctress sprinkled the breast of the infant with water, using her right hand, with a prayer for long life and health of the child; and, dipping her hand into the vase of water, she proceeded to bathe the child. After the bath the child's entire body was rubbed over with ashes. The cloth which had previously wrapped the infant was changed for another, which, however, was neither new nor clean. A blanket that had been previously warmed by the fire was afterward placed around the child. The young mother observed the bathing and wrapping of her infant with great interest. The infant was next laid upon a fresh sand bed prepared by the paternal grandmother, and the young mother walked to her bed and lay down, while a doctress bathed the lacerated perineum with warm root tea and afterward sprinkled the affected parts with a powder,[6] after which she manipulated the abdomen for thirty minutes. The young mother then sat upon the ledge by the fire while a fresh sand bed was prepared for her. After a time the child was placed to the breast, but it failed to get nourishment, though it made persistent effort. The hot juniper tea was drunk constantly after the confinement for the purpose of hastening the close of the lochial discharge, which ceased after the fourth day. On the second day, October 22, the pulse of the mother was seventy-eight. Though several efforts were made through the day to nourish the child from the mother, the milk did not appear. On the twenty-third the pulse was seventy-nine. Mother and child were doing well. The lacerated

5. The Zuñis declare that in four days from the putting on of the ashes exfoliation occurs and a new skin appears. Ashes are used throughout the first year to render the face and other parts of the body depilous. With rare exceptions, these people are depilous, except on the scalp.
6. In aggravated cases of laceration certain male theurgists are called in. In the case here mentioned the parts appeared to be entirely healed after the eighth day. The tea and powder were used only four days. The powder secured by the writer was not of sufficient quantity to admit an analysis.

perineum was much improved. The same treatment was continued. Though the feet and ankles were excessively swollen for days before parturition, they rapidly returned to their normal condition after the birth of the child. On the twenty-fourth the pulse was seventy-nine. Though the milk came, it appeared like pus, and the child refused it. The infant was so weak from lack of nourishment that the writer prepared condensed milk, upon which it was fed for some days, and its improvement was marked. On the twenty-fifth the pulse was ninety. The infant was placed to the breast several times, but refused the milk. At the first light of day on the twenty-sixth, a line of meal, symbolic of the path of life, was sprinkled from the house to the point where the child was to observe for the first time the Sun Father. The doctress who had received the child when it came into the world, accompanied by the young mother and the paternal grandmother, carried the infant, with the ear of corn which had been by its side since its birth held close to its head. The doctress stooped and held the child to face east while she offered a prayer for the health and happiness, goodness of heart, and long life of the child. At sunrise the doctress dipped up several gourdfuls of water in which juniper had been steeped and emptied it into a bowl near the fireplace; then the paternal great-grandmother of the child poured yucca root and handed it to the doctress, who made suds of it by beating it in the juniper water. As the bowl became filled with snowy froth, she took off the suds, putting them into a second bowl, and when this bowl was filled, the suds were warmed with hot juniper water. The paternal grandmother held the child until the doctress had removed her moccasins and was seated on a blanket spread on the floor. The physician held the infant, its head to the east, supporting it with the left hand. The great-grandmother and the paternal grandmother stood one on each side of the bowl. The doctress first dipped a handful of suds, and then the others took suds with their right hands. The young mother sat on the ledge nearby, but took no part. The suds were held while the doctress offered a long prayer to A'wonawil'ona, the Sun Father, and the Earth Mother, that all blessings might come to the child. At the conclusion of the prayer the doctress placed the suds she held on the top of the child's head, and then the other two patted the suds on the head; and the head was then held over the bowl and thoroughly washed by the doctress. Great care was observed in bathing the eyes; they were smoothed over and over, and the nose was pinched many times. A blanket was folded and spread over the extended legs of the doctress, in the manner heretofore described, a wad being placed before the upturned feet where the child's head was to rest. The dressing was removed from the umbilicus, which was found entirely healed. The child was then bathed from a bowl containing only warm juniper water. The paternal grandmother was careful to warm the cloths in which the child was to be wrapped. Nothing was used to dry the child aside from the ashes which were rubbed over its entire body. The infant, still refusing its mother's milk, was fed with condensed milk from a spoon. It smacked its lips with satisfaction, much to the delight of the paternal grandfather and the others present. The child was then held by the grandmother, while the doctress worked up anew the yucca suds. The young mother's hair was loosed, and she bent her head over the bowl while the doctress, the mother-in-law, and the latter's mother and young niece dipped suds with their right hands and held them while the doctress prayed. After the prayer the doctress applied to the head the suds she held, and the others did the same, after which the doctress thoroughly washed the head and long hair. The young mother then took her seat while the doctress removed the remainder of her sand bed, which was carried in a blanket to the far end of the room and deposited in a heap. The doctress afterward placed by the sand heap the bowl of juniper water, in which the yucca suds had been deposited to bathe the infant, and proceeded to bathe the young mother, who was now at the other end of the room. The girl kept on her camis, which soon became thoroughly wet. The doctress poured water over her by the gourdful. The girl washed her own legs, standing while she did so. Twenty minutes were consumed in this bath, though the large room, except near the fire, was very cold. No cloth was used to dry the body. A soiled camis was slipped on her as she dropped the other, and, wrapping a heavy blanket around herself, the young mother walked over the cold stone floor in her bare feet, which were still swollen, and took her seat by the fire. Within twenty minutes after the bath the mother's pulse was eighty-two. She seemed perfectly well and declared that she felt so. An excellent meal was served, but the grandfather was too absorbed to leave his work of attaching buckskin thongs and loops to the new cradle, which was a present from the paternal uncle Mauretio. On the cradle, just where the head of the infant should rest, was a perfectly round turquoise of excellent color. Inlaid below and close to the neck rest were three turquoises. When the cradle was completed, the child was strapped to it. In folding the wraps around the child care was observed first to bring around the piece of cotton from the right side of the child so as to prevent the arms from coming in contact with the body, the cloth passing under each arm. The other side of the cloth was then brought over both arms. The blanket was folded around and tied in two places. On the twenty-seventh the mother's pulse was eighty-two.

She was sitting up, dressed, and apparently perfectly well. The infant took the mother's milk for the first time. The pulse was the same on the twenty-eighth and twenty-ninth. The mother was up and sewing on the twenty-ninth, and the child took much notice and appeared brighter and more observing than any civilized child of the same age known to the writer.

—*Matilda C. Stevenson*

56: The Trauma of Birth

For nine months the child lives and grows in the quiet contentment of its mother's womb. Without struggle or effort, all its wants are gratified. The sense of perpetuity with which its requirements are taken care of makes the child feel like a God in a universe of its own. Nothing comes to it in overwhelming abundance or in frustrating meagerness. Conditions for its development are ideal. The eternity of the fetal night knows of no breaks. The idea of change is beyond conception. Growth is a sensation giving strength and power. It not only leaves the child's environment unaltered, but enhances the feeling of omnipotence which the perfection of its environment inspires. The existence of an overshadowing, all-enveloping Supreme Being called Mother, the awe-inspiring reality of a vast outer universe peopled with incomprehensible giants are infinitely removed from the cosmos of the tiny God of the Womb.

Suddenly, in an apocalyptic upheaval, its instinctive awareness is trampled in the dust, its sensation of power is crushed; an abyss opens under the very foundations of its universe; and in the awful drama of birth the God that the child was discovers pain and fear. We cannot picture the bewilderment which these strange new sensations bring in their wake. We can only trace their origin from what we know about the physiology of birth.

The rumblings of the approaching end of the fetal kingdom strike the child in the same way that primitive people are stricken by an earthquake or a tidal wave from the sea. The rock and the earth begin to move from under them; water bursts over their shore dwellings. They are confronted by a cataclysm presaging the end of their world.

Instead of a tidal wave, the ordeal of the child about to be born begins by the sudden ebbing away of the waters of birth. The amniotic fluid that cushions the child and safeguards it from the shocks caused by movements of the mother's body (or her falling accidents) begins to recede, whereupon contractions of the mother's ejectory muscles raise the curtain to the perilous journey to life. Compared to an unborn babe's power of resistance, this constitutes an earthquake. The breaking of the birth waters and the beginning of labor are not always closely linked. In cases of accident, the amniotic sac may burst days before, in which event the mother must be confined to her bed in order to avoid premature birth.

The loss of the waters is the first violent and unwelcome change in the prenatal environment. It produces tactile reactions for which the child is not prepared. Of the five human senses, only the sense of touch operates in the prenatal state. It is stimulated by a contact of the child's limbs with its own body, by the buoyancy of the amniotic fluid and by the feel, through the caul, of the fleshy folds of the walls of the uterus. An early loss of the waters deprives the child of the delightful sensation of floating (the memories of which we often recapture in swimming and flying dreams) and restricts the ease and comfort of its movements. The contact with the maternal environment becomes rough and irritating, and the mother's movements in bed may register as minor collisions.

In the course of birth the lower part of the uterus dilates under the constant pressure of muscles that contract on the body of the child, holding it in an iron grip. A hormone substance softens the mother's tissues and bones to permit necessary dilatation for the passing of the child. As a rule the child is in a headfirst position. If not, birth cannot take place in the usual manner. The child may have to be pushed back and turned by instruments. Its skin, already sorely tried by the ejectory shocks and the pressure against the pubic arch, is too delicate to be unaffected by the forceps, however skillfully handled. Severe bruising may result. After this kind of delivery, the child may scream for a day or two upon being touched. The bruises tell their own tale. Neurotics who have a morbid fear of being touched may suffer from the unreleased psychic pressure of the tactile shocks suffered in birth or prior to it from the loss of the amniotic fluid.

The beginning of the mother's labor is the second violent change in the prenatal environment. Hitherto this environment was friendly and beneficent; now it appears hostile. When labor is prolonged, in the absence of consciousness of the purpose of the process, the child goes through an agony only comparable to the slow torture of death. There is no intellectual acceptance as in the case of the mother to mitigate the pain and terror of the experience. The mother knows she is not likely to die; the child does not. The mother may be helped by twilight sleep, which will also affect the child. The child may be born asleep. But the drug bars the pain and shock from consciousness only, and not from the organism itself. The unborn child is nothing but an organism. Unconscious as it may be, the pain and fear reactions will still register. It is possible, however, that sleep produced during the most critical period of delivery helps to develop the mechanism of repression. It is a moot question, though, whether such repression should be encouraged. It may make the release of the trauma of birth more difficult and thereby, in the long run, contribute to neurosis.

The third violent change in the prenatal environment is the actual birth. During the prenatal state the child is supplied with oxygen through the mother's blood, which reaches its system by way of the umbilical cord. The breathing apparatus is fully developed at seven months, but it does not begin to function until after birth. During the mother's labor, the child still receives its oxygen supply through the cord, but on leaving the maternal body the cord detaches itself from its mooring in the placenta and trails along attached to the navel of the child. As it no longer carries blood and oxygen, a time interval ensues before pulmonary activity begins. Some babies cry lustily as soon as they are born. The cry means that the lungs have started functioning without external stimulation. Other babies, however, turn blue immediately after birth and are in danger of death from suffocation. When the doctor turns them upside down and slaps them on the buttocks, their lungs start working. These late breathers go through another shock—the sensation of air pressure on an uninflated chest. Morbid suffocation fears in later life may often be traced to such delayed breathing. Occasionally the delay is due to accidents. The umbilical cord may be wound around the child's neck and obstruct breathing until it is removed.

Reaction to the doctor's slap is sometimes shown in birth dreams. A young woman, in the course of dramatically reliving her birth on the analyst's couch, described the doctor's slap as "flames of light flaring up in my brain." The seat of pain is in the brain. Only by training do we learn to localize the sensation at the nerve endings from which the stimulus of pain started. Immediately after birth this training is absent. "Flames of light in the brain" is not only a vivid description of the nerve reactions of the newborn child but suggests that birth injuries veritably set the child's brain on fire.

The behaviorist school of psychology claims that there are two original fears, not acquired but born with us: the fear of loss of position and the fear of loud sounds. The behaviorists mean that both fears are part of our instinctual heritage because they are present from birth without any accounting for them. I am not in accord with this view. The fear of loss of position is acquired. It originates in the pushes the child experiences from the contractions of the ejectory muscles. The child is head-downward in the uterus and falls away from its post on being born. Most abnormal fears of falling can be traced to the fall from the uterine heaven into the terrestrial abyss. The legend of the Fall of Man is a record of our biological origin.

—Nandor Fodor

57: My Mother's Womb

My first house
It was all around
Sometimes I wonder
What I was like then

Feet against your heart mama
Knees tight to your liver
Hands shrunk to the tube
That ties to your womb

My back swivelled
Ears filled up my eyes empty
All of me curled up taut twisted
My head almost out of your belly

Thin skull at your opening
I had all of your health
The heat of your blood
And papa's holding you

Sometimes a hybrid fire
Electrified my darkness
A knock at my skull unwound me
I rushed at your heart

Your cunt's great muscle
Tightened around me, painfully

I let it be done to me with sorrow
You poured blood down all around me

My forehead's still dented
From those hard thrusts of father
Why did it have to be done to me
Half-strangled inside you?

If I could have opened my mouth
I would have gnawed at you
If I could have spoken then
I would have shouted

Shit—I don't want to live!
—*Blaise Cendrars*

58: Delivery Songs

Songs used at the time of delivery are again rare. In the Chattisgarh plain there is no taboo, as there is among the wilder tribes, on the employment of midwives. The songs refer to the knife to cut the umbilical cord, the pot used for the mother's bath of purification, and the "flower" or placenta, which is buried in a pit, sometimes in the actual place of birth, sometimes outside the house.

Many methods are used to accelerate a difficult delivery, and many have been recorded. Two that are, I think, new may be mentioned here. A Brahmin gave a Gond woman a railway ticket, telling her to wash it and drink the water, whereupon she would be delivered with the speed of a train. A Pardhan who had been married three times was in some demand, for the water in which the feet of so adventurous a traveller had been washed was regarded as very efficacious.

1.
The sun is red in the sky
The crows are talking
Call the midwife
For my darling is weary
My body is tormented with pain
Call the midwife quickly
My darling is tired of the dark
He is fighting to escape.

2.
Father-in-law is asleep in the yard
Mother-in-law is asleep on the verandah
My little dewar is in his colored palace
Wake wake sister-in-law

Tell my child's father
There is pain in my belly
Send for the midwife
My sweet baby is coming
The knife is of gold
The pot is of silver
The flower is a rose
Or is it a lotus?
The cord is cut
The flower is buried
Deep deep is the pit
My sweet baby is crying.

> The "little dewar" is the husband's younger brother, with whom a traditional
> intimacy is permitted: the reference here may mean that he is the child's real
> father. The knife is to cut the cord; the pot is for the ceremonial bath; the
> flower is the placenta; the pit in which it is buried must be deep, for should a
> witch steal it or an animal dig it up, it would be disastrous for the child.

3.
Lallu's born, Lallu's born
Run boy and get the midwife
What knife shall we use to cut the cord?
What pot shall we use for the bath?
With a golden knife we will cut the cord
With a silver pot we will bathe.

4.
A son is born today, brother
A son is born today
In their best clothes my wife's friends are coming
When my wife's son was born
The pain scorched her body
A son is born today, brother
A son is born today.

I called the barber and washerman
They soon did their work
Daily the child grew bigger
And my life was filled with joy
Blessed be my wife's body

Though her loins were undone with pain
I watch her night and day
A son is born today, brother
A son is born today.

5.
In the early morning a son was born
Jagat Raja has gone to sleep
Before the midwife will cut the cord
She demands a present in Neng
She has taken my nose-ring in Neng
Jagat Raja has gone to sleep
Before the barber will cut the hair
He demands a present in Neng
He has taken my anklets in Neng
Jagat Raja has gone to sleep
Before the washerman will wash the clothes
He demands a present in Neng
He has taken my red sari in Neng.

> The word Neng covers a social custom and an attitude of mind that is
> characteristic of this part of India. On all ceremonial occasions—it may be
> birth, marriage, festival, funeral—certain privileged persons, relatives, or
> officials of the rite, hold up the proceedings and demand a present. Nothing
> can proceed until the ceremonial tax is paid. This is a fruitful source of dispute
> in weddings, for on such occasions there are many relatives to be bought off.
> Here, after the birth of a child, the midwife, barber, and washerman refuse to
> fulfill their proper functions until they are given their proper dues. This is
> Neng, a word of great importance for the understanding of the Chattisgarhi
> mind.

—Verrier Elwin

59: Tale of How an Old Woman Induced Delivery

The remarkable Arnold of Villanova (c. 1235–1311), a Spanish physician who was also a lawyer, theologian, and philosopher, discusses obstetrical problems at some length and tells a quaint tale about the method which "a certain old woman of Salerno" swore was nearly always successful in inducing a delivery. The old woman used three grains of pepper:

> With each grain she said one paternoster. When she should have said, "Deliver us from evil," she said instead, "Deliver this woman, O Mary, from this difficult labor." Then she gave her the three grains to swallow, one after another, with wine or water with the instruction that none of the three grains be touched with the teeth. Then she said these words three times with three paternosters in her right ear: "Bizomie: lamion: lamium: azerai vachina Lord. Lord of sabaoth. Sky and earth are full of thy glory. Hosanna in the highest." With these words in her ears, the woman delivered at once.

Arnold adds sternly, "I deprecate all this and believe that all the faithful should shun such diabolical practices and remedies."

60: How An Unborn Child Avenged Its Mother's Death

A man had taken a wife, and now she had the joy of being with child, but famine was acute in the land.

One day, when hunger was particularly severe, the man, accompanied by his wife, was dragging himself along in the direction of her mother's home in the hope of getting a little food there. He happened to find on the road a tree with abundant wild fruit on the top. "Wife," he said "get up there that we may eat fruit."

The woman refused, saying, "I, who am with child, to climb up a tree!"

He said, "In that case, do not climb at all."

The husband then climbed up himself and shook and shook the branches, the woman meanwhile picking up what fell down. He said, "Do not pick up my fruit. What! Just now you refused to go up!"

And she: "*Bana!* I am only picking them up."

Thinking about his fruit, he hurried down from the top of the tree and said, "You have eaten some."

And she: "Why! Of course, I have not."

Then, assegai in hand, he stabbed his wife. And there she died on the spot.

He then gathered up his fruit with both hands. There he sat eating it, remaining where the woman was stretched out quite flat.

All of a sudden he started running. Run! Run! Run! Without stopping once, he ran until he reached the rise of a hill.

There he slept, out of sight of the place where he had left the woman.

Meanwhile the child that was in the womb rushed out of it, dragging its umbilical cord. First, it looked round for the direction which its father had taken, then it started this song:

Father, wait for me,
Father, wait for me,
The little wombless.

Who is it that has eaten my mother?
The little wombless . . .!
How swollen are those eyes!
Wait till the little wombless comes.

That gave the man a shake. . . . "There," he said, "there comes the thing which is speaking." He listened, he stared in that direction. . . . "This is the child coming to follow me after all that, when I have already killed its mother. It had been left in the womb."

Then rage took his wits away, and he killed the little child! . . . There he was, making a fresh start, and going on. Here, where the little bone had been left: "Little bone, gather yourself up! . . . Little bone, gather yourself up."

Soon it was up again, and then came the song:

Father wait for me,
Father, wait for me,
The little wombless
Who is it that has eaten my mother?
The little wombless . . . !
How swollen are those eyes!
Wait till the little wombless comes.

The father stopped. . . . "Again the child that I have killed! It has risen and is coming. Now I shall wait for him."

So he hid and waited for the child, with an assegai in his hand. The child came and made itself visible at a distance as from here to there. As soon as it came, quick with the assegai! He stabbed it! Then he looked for a hole, shoveled the little body into it, and heaped branches up at the entrance.

Then with all speed he ran! With all speed! . . .

At last he reached the kraal where the mother of his dead wife lived, the grandmother of the child.

When he came he sat down. Then his brothers and sisters-in-law come with smiling faces. . . . "Well! Well! You have put in an appearance!"

"We have," he says, "put in an appearance."

And a hut was prepared for him and his wife, who was expected.

Then the mother-in-law was heard asking from afar, "Well! And my daughter, where has she been detained?"

Said he, "I have left her at home. I have come alone to beg for a little food. Hunger is roaring."

"Sit down inside there, father."

Food was procured for him. So he began to eat. And, when he had finished, he even went to sleep.

Meanwhile, the child, on its part, had squeezed itself out of the hole wherein it had been put and, again, with its umbilical cord hanging on:

Father, wait for me,
Father, wait for me,
The little wombless.
Who is it that has eaten my mother?
The little wombless . . .!
How swollen are those eyes!
Wait till the little wombless comes.

The people listened in the direction of the path. . . . "That thing which comes speaking indistinctly, what is it? . . . It seems to be a person. . . . What is it? . . . It looks, man, like a child killed by you on the road. . . . And now, when we look at your way of sitting, you seem to be only half-seated."

"It cannot be the child, Mother; it remained at home." The man had just got up to shake himself a little. And his little child, too, was coming with all speed! It was already near, with its mouth wide open:

Father, wait for me,
Father, wait for me,
The little wombless.
Who is it that has eaten my mother?
The little wombless . . .!
How swollen are those eyes!
Wait till the little wombless comes!

Everyone was staring. They said, "There comes a little red thing. It still has the umbilical cord hanging on."

Inside of the hut there, where the man stood, there was complete silence!

Meanwhile the child was coming on feet and buttocks with its mouth wide open, but still at a distance from its grandmother's hut. "Straight over there!" noted everyone. The grandmother looked toward the road and noticed that the little thing was perspiring, and what speed! Then the song:

Father, wait for me,
Father, wait for me,
The little wombless.
Who is it that has eaten my mother?
The little wombless . . .!
Who is it that has eaten my mother?
The little wombless . . .!
How swollen are those eyes!
Wait till the little wombless comes.

Bakoo! It scarcely reached its grandmother's hut when it jumped into it . . . and up on the bed:

> Father, wait for me,
> Father, have you come?
> Yes, you have eaten my mother.
> How swollen those eyes!
> Wait till the little wombless comes.

Then the grandmother put this question to the man: "Now what sort of song is this child singing? Have you not killed our daughter?"

She had scarcely added, "Surround him!" when he was already in their hands. His very brothers-in-law tied him. And then . . . all the assegais were poised together in one direction, everyone saying, "Now today you are the man who killed our sister. . . ."

Then they just threw the body away there to the west. And the grandmother picked up her little grandchild.

—Bena Mukuni

61: Siberian Childbirth Ceremonies

As soon as a woman notices signs of pregnancy (*pōjtas* in the Mansi language means literally "something has discontinued"), she starts to observe the strict rules of conduct which govern that condition. For instance, in the fourth to fifth months of pregnancy she must possess a *sōs*[1] which she makes herself if she can, or which is made by some other woman with dextrous hands, who is considered an expert in making such [a] doll. But the maker must not be a female shaman.

Preparing the *sōs* is a process which is concealed from strangers; it is connected with a feast. The person who prepares the *sōs* interrupts her work at various stages to pray and eat, and then resumes work, or turns to the religious consecration of the doll. When the doll is ready, a string of glass beads is hung around its neck and braids are fixed in the back. The waist is girded with a ribbon the ends of which hang loose at the back. The doll is held by means of this ribbon when necessary, so that it stays in a vertical position. The *sōs* is meant for the *šāń*[2] "mother" and establishes a connection between the mother and the *šāń*. If the woman has a *sōs*, the child will not be too big and the delivery will be easier.

The *sōs* is kept in the woman's *tutšaŋ*[3] neatly wrapped up in a pretty shawl or in the skin of some small wild animal. Later on this is presented as a gift to the *pupiyšáŋ*.

Usually in the fifth or sixth month of her pregnancy the woman builds a very primitive cradle (*ampten sán*)[4] in which the infant sleeps for the

1. *sōs* — a female figurine as big as the thumb. It is made from the soft dried brown growth of the birch tree.
2. *šáń* — a *pupiy* which is represented as a grey-haired woman who is believed to send the children who are supposed to be born. When she is not angry with the future mother, she sends a boy; otherwise, a girl.
3. *tutšaŋ* — a pretty little bag which is decorated with beads, ornaments, chamois colored fringes, used for holding sewing accessories.
4. *ampten sán* — (literally: a cup of birch bark for the feeding of dogs) a primitive cradle, made of birch bark. It looks like a trough.

first week of its life. A small warm coverlet (*léŋkw*) of swan skin or the winter fur of a hare, as well as a small pillow, *sasnétmil*,[5] made of the soft fur of deer, etc., are also provided for.

For herself the woman prepares a very shabby garment and a pair of old shoes which she will wear during the first week after the delivery (later on this dress will be hung on a tree in the woods, or will be exposed in a birch bark bucket, in a part of the forest which is never visited by people). She also weaves a *tówar*,[6] on which she will sit and sleep. All these things are kept ready for use and strictly hidden from the sight of men and strangers.

During the nine months of pregnancy the expectant mother herself, or some other woman who does not belong to the family, takes the *sōs* in her arms from time to time, kisses it and holds it in a perpendicular position by the ends of the ribbon with the tips of three fingers. The woman who is holding the *sōs* must divine whether the expectant mother will live through the birth, whether the child will be healthy, etc. This is revealed from the way the *sōs* moves. It is an auspicious sign if it swings smoothly and quietly; whereas if it hangs motionless or twitches, something unfavorable must be expected. The *sōs* must be taken more frequently in hand as the time of birth approaches.

Just before confinement, the mother goes to live in the *māṅkol*. She takes along the *tutšāŋ* and the other objects which she has prepared for the event. In the small house she removes her good clothes, and puts on the old ones. Then she or one of the women makes a fire in the *šowal*,[7] boils water and prepares flat stones with which to keep her body warm after the birth of the child. (During the delivery not only the close relatives who assist the woman but also girls over ten years of age are permitted to watch the patient and to share with her the labor pains. The girls are told: "Obey your mother! Look at the pain with which she brought you into this world!")

To facilitate the delivery a special apparatus is made. Two parallel vertical rods are set up about one meter from each other; their ends are firmly attached to the floor and to the ceiling, and then a crossbar is fixed to them at a height of seventy centimeters. At critical moments the

---

5. *sansnétmil*—a sheet of birch wood, about twice the size of the palm of a hand. It is laid on the knees of the child together with a reindeer skin to prevent its feet from becoming crooked, and the blanket from getting wet.

6. *tówar*—a mattress made of bundles of long dry grass (with strings).

7. *šowal*—chimney for the fireplace which is usually in the right corner of the house, facing the door. It is made in the following way: thin vertical poles are placed next to each other in order to form a large-diameter tube; their ends are bound together and they are smudged with a thick layer of clay mixed with a soft grass called *wānsi*.

woman leans with her breast against the rods and supports herself by her armpits.

In the case of a difficult or late delivery one of the women takes the *sōs* in her hands to find out what the trouble is and whether the child will soon appear. In this manner the woman may discover that the reason for the difficulties or for the delay might be improper language which the woman has sometimes used in connection with somebody, or a husband's love affair with another woman during the pregnancy of his wife, or previous infidelity of the woman who is in labor. If the husband is found guilty, one of the women goes immediately from the *mānkol* to the big house and tells him that his wife cannot recover and that *he* is to blame for it. If he does not wish his wife to suffer or to die, he must at once confess how many times, and with whom, he has betrayed his wife during her pregnancy. With this information the woman hastens back to the *mānkol* and makes one notch on one of the vertical rods for each time the woman has been deceived, according tó the confession of the husband. If the patient herself is to blame, the woman turns to her and then makes one notch on the other vertical rod for each time she has committed adultery. By this method the infidelity of both the husband and the wife is revealed.

During the confinement the husband must stay at home in the big house and wait for the child to be born.

The expectant mother customarily hangs her most beautiful kerchief on the front corner of the *mānkol,* for the *šāń.* The female shaman *ńājt-nē*[8] informs the *šāń* of its presence there. If the patient's condition is serious, the strongest male shaman is called for. He proceeds as follows: He takes an axe in his hands and binds a string to the axe and to its handle so that the axe is hanging with its edge upwards. Then he turns to some *pupiy* in his thoughts and with the aid of the axe he discovers the cause of the woman's pains and states what kind of sacrifice is necessary. In extreme cases, the shaman prepares a *turmankol.*[9] Sometimes it is revealed to him that a certain *pupiy,* or *ten-ajn-kuľ*[10] demands the patient herself as the sacrifice. It is believed that the shaman has the power to save her life by indicating somebody else, a complete stranger. This innocent person may die soon after the substitution. The shamans

8. *ńājt-nē* — a female shaman. She carries a thin and slender piece of board, the length of a finger, fixes the end of a knife to it, then lifts the board and sits waiting for the swaying of the suspended knife.
9. *turmankol* — (literally: "dark house"). The shaman works at night in the house, which is completely dark, either alone or in the presence of many people. He finds out the cause of the illness in a conversation with the *pupiy* by means of a musical instrument called *sāŋkwoltap.*
10. *ten-ajn-kuľ* — something infernal, having invisible spiritual existence.

were greatly feared by the simple people because of this "power" of theirs. They used to boast that they would send to the other world any person who would refuse to pay due respect to them.

When the child is born there is general rejoicing. One of the women cuts the *pùkńi,* the placenta. When this is done, the child's face is smeared with blood so that the child will have red cheeks later on. The placenta is then tied down and the wound is sprinkled with dust from a corner of the hut. The woman who has cut the *pùkńi* will be addressed by the child later as *pùkńišān* (literally: "navel mother"), and she, in turn, calls the child *pùkńipiy,* or *pùkńiāyi* (literally: "navel son" or "navel daughter"). The child's mother must present this woman with a knife, and sometimes also with other objects. The *pùkńišān* washes the child and puts it into the cradle which has been supplied by the mother. Then a meal is prepared with which the birth of the child is celebrated for the first and last time.

The dress of the mother must be torn down in the front from top to bottom so that it becomes a gown. This happens because the Mansi say that the child dropped out through the belly and tore the dress. (After the birth of the child the mother wears a girdle which is made of hair to help her body regain its normal shape.)

Dressed in her worst clothes for one week, the mother must run out in the street, exposed to the cold in the winter, and to the mosquitoes in the summer. With this the first phase of purification is over,[11] and the woman may change her clothes for better ones. But she is not through with the ordeal yet: she has to undress in the frost, or expose her body to legions of mosquitoes, which finally purify her. (The same method is resorted to during menstruation at any arbitrary place such as in a wood, on a road, etc.)

At the end of the first week the mother cleans the child of the invisible "impurity" which is believed to have been transferred to it from her. For the purification of the child the *sōs* made for the *šāń,* as well as its *lālwa,*[12] is used. Then the child is put to sleep in another cradle, or in another bed. The mother's old dress and the child's first cradle are carried to the woods and hidden in the most "impure" spot, behind the *māńkol,* where all the first cradles of the children who are born in that *māńkol* are hung up. The *šāń-pājup*[13] (literally: "the mother's basket") is also hung up on the branch of a tree, as high as possible. If the child is to live long, the basket must remain hanging there for a long time.

11. *taktalaytil* — the process of getting rid of the invisible "impurity."
12. *lālwa* — a dried piece of castor, i.e., a musk bag of the beaver.
13. *šāń-pājup* — an improvised cover of birch bark in which the placenta is placed.

It is not until three months after the childbirth that the woman decides to make preparations for her return to the big house. For this purpose she must go through careful purification ceremonies to free herself from invisible "impurity:" she makes a *sāpjiv-χāp*[14] and adorns it with little rings which are made from very thin twigs. In the middle she makes a little hole, into which she lays the *sōs* (a piece of dry brown birch wood), lights it and places on it the *lālwa,* which emits a special "purifying" odor as it burns. The water in which the child and the mother are washed is prepared in a special manner. While it is being warmed, the burnt *sōs* is thrown in, then it is grated into powder in the water and then dissolved. The water changes slightly its color and becomes soft and velvety. A piece of chewed *lālwa,* which mixes with it and dissolves, is thrown into the water, obviously for the purpose of rendering it more sacred. As soon as the water has settled, the woman washes herself first and then the child. When she is clean, she puts on her clothes. Then she lays on a stone a red-hot axe which steams and causes a hissing sound when it gets into contact with the moist *ossi* which have been thrown on it. With her child and with all things that were with her in the *māṅkol,* the woman jumps over the steam shouting "*kuχ-kuχ,*" thereby getting rid of her load of "impurity," which is carried away by the steam. When this has been done, she takes the *sāpjiv-χāp* in which the smoldering *sōs* lies with the *lālwa.* The smell of the *lālwa* spreads through the whole house. The woman begins to carry the *sāpjiv-χāp* all over the *māṅkol* holding it under objects and chairs. The smoke and smell of the *sōs* and *lālwa* clean away the last remains of "impurity." Later the woman holds also the child in the cradle over this little boat and steps over it several times herself. At last she is completely "clean." She can now go into the big house, yet not before one more ceremony has been performed: one of the women takes the child together with the cradle, which is covered with a beautiful kerchief, while the mother grasps the *tutšaŋ* in one hand and the *sāpjiv-χāp* in the other. Then having made one first step, they stop and put the *sāpjiv-χāp* on the floor over which the woman with the child jumps first, then the mother, saying: "*šanttiy-ponttiy.*" (The meaning of these two words is not quite clear.) They now go out of the *māṅkol,* but on the way to the big house the same ceremony is repeated several times.

When they reach the house the woman who is carrying the child

14. *sāpjiv-χap* — this looks like a toy ship made of rotted birch or willow which easily yields to the woman's knife.

knocks at the door and says: "Hi! open the door, the woman (man) has arrived on four reindeer, on five reindeer," or "the woman who owns horses, who owns cows has arrived." Thereupon she opens the door a little with her elbow and shows the child, with its feet forward; then she closes the door again. This is repeated four times if the child is a girl, and five times in case it is a boy. Finally the woman flings the door open and jumps with the child into the house, saying: "*šanttiy-ponttiy*." Then the child is carried to the front corner where the cradle is set up. To celebrate the arrival of the child in the house, a feast is arranged.

The woman who carried the child to the house is from now on called *altumšáń* (literally: "mother by carrying"). The kerchief with which the child was covered is given to the *altumšáń* as a present. The ribbon or string, which was placed on the knees of the child when it was brought to the big house, and pierced with four needles in the case of a girl and with five in the case of a boy, is also presented to this woman. The needles represent skunks. Later also the *altumšáń* has to present her *altumáyi* (literally: "daughter by carrying") with a gift.

Besides the *pùkńišáń* and *altumšáń* the child must have also a *pernaŋšáń* ("godfather"); and a *pernaŋáš* ("godmother") who usually give crosses to the child and expect to receive a present. No christening ceremony is performed.

It is believed that some time after the birth of the child the soul of a dead person whose will to live has been strong moves into it, i.e., the child "clashes with it" (in Mansi *ľaχiχati*).[15] The souls of one or several dead persons may move into the body of a newborn child. A dead man may transmit his soul five times to children who are born at different times; a woman may transmit hers four times, because a woman has four souls whereas a man has five.

The soul of a dead person is believed to enter the child when it begins to cry at night. It is supposed to be disturbed by something or somebody. At daytime when it is sleeping, it is carefully moved with the cradle; then somebody—usually one of the women—lifts it carefully while thinking of one of the dead relatives. If the child becomes suddenly very heavy they have found out who troubled it and it will stop crying.

If a child is stillborn or dies during the first week of its life, it is not buried in the common cemetery, but in the dry soil of a completely

---

15. *ľaχtχattuŋkwe* (possibly from the word *ľeŋntχatunkwe*) "clash against one another," as the soul of the dead person against the child.

isolated pine forest. When a commemoration service is held for the child, no bonfire is lit at the grave but warm food is brought from the house. This divergence from the normal funeral repasts, where everything is prepared on bonfires in the cemetery, is due to the belief that the child, being so small, can neither light a bonfire nor eat anything warm.

— E. I. Rombandeeva

VI Events After Birth, Naming, Baptizing

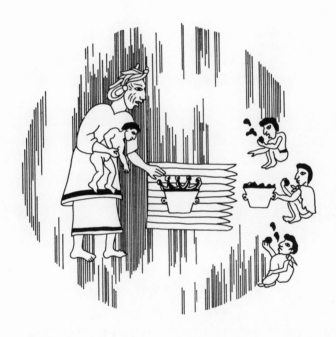

Infant Joy

"I have no name;
I am but two days old."
What shall I call thee?
"I happy am;
Joy is my name."
— Sweet joy befall thee!

Pretty joy!
Sweet joy, but two days old;
Sweet joy I call thee:
Thou dost smile:
I sing the while,
Sweet joy befall thee!
          — William Blake

62: "Water Has Been Put on Top of His Head"

A few days after birth a major rite is conducted which further associates the child with his family and with the protective supernaturals.

> There is a ceremony of the earth which is a long-life ceremony.[1] Every child goes through this. The gods gave the people this ceremony in the beginning. It is handed down from old times through the tribe. This ceremony was given to the people when they were already on this earth, before Monster Slayer came, however, and before the monsters were killed.[2] It was not needed for life in the underworld before the emergence, for down there, there was no sickness, no death, no need for a long-life ceremony like this. But the earth is dangerous and evil; and this takes the children to the puberty ceremony safely.[3]

The name of the ceremony is "water has been put on top of his head." It always takes place the fourth day after birth. Even if the mother is not well enough to stand up for the ceremony, it has to go on. In that case she lies down. They get someone who knows the songs to sing them for the baby. My father and S— and my father-in-law know this ceremony; J— knows it too. The man is paid according to what the family wants to give him; no certain things have to be given.

The child has not been washed before: this is the first time since birth that water has touched it. They do not use the water from springs or

1. The principal Jicarilla ceremonies are those which have their justification in the myths and which have existed "from the beginning." They can be learned and perpetuated by those who are pious and industrious enough to seek instruction from persons who already know them. Shamanistic ceremonies, or those which begin with a personal supernatural experience and a power grant, exist, but they are less important and are not nearly so elaborate or so well-considered as the long-life ceremonies.
2. Monster Slayer, as his name suggests, is the leading culture hero of the Jicarilla. He aided the tribe during the mythological period when its existence was threatened by monsters. The story of the slaying of these monsters is an integral part of Jicarilla mythology. See Opler, *Myths and Tales of the Jicarilla Apache Indians*, pp. 57–77.
3. According to their sacred legend, the Jicarilla, before they emerged upon this earth, lived in darkness in the underworld. When the sun and the moon were created, boastful

lakes when they have this ceremony. They use the water from rivers. It has to be from the sacred male rivers, the Arkansas and the Rio Grande, and the sacred female rivers, the Pecos and the Canadian. When they first get the water they offer sacred stones, such as turquoise and red beads, to the rivers. Water from at least one of the male rivers and one of the female rivers must be mixed together. The one who has charge and is going to sing gets the water.

The singer starts early, before the sun comes up. He puts the water in a clay bowl.[4] He sprinkles pollen sunwise in the form of a sun on top of the water. Then he does the same with specular iron ore and he makes four rays of pollen and specular iron ore extending outward to the directions, beginning with the east. Then he brings grama grass and snakeweed. Grama grass is used by all the holy people, like the gods. It is leader for the growing things, for the plants. Snakeweed is another holy one that is much used in the ceremonies and therefore has its place here. The singer puts grama grass in the water with the top part up. Then he crushes the snakeweed and puts in pieces from the inside of the plant top.

He now starts to sing about the pollen and the specular iron ore. He sings for long life for the child. He sings of those four rivers, because those rivers have long life, and we people live by means of water. He is holding the naked child in his hands. He dips his right hand in the water and sprinkles water four times on the baby's right foot. Then he does it to the right hand of the child, to the right shoulder, then to the top of the head, to the left shoulder, to the left hand, and to the left foot.

Now he washes the feet of the child with the water and works right up the baby's body to the head. Next he sprinkles water on the baby's blanket and on what is prepared for the baby's diaper. Now he is finished with the water. It is thrown four times to the east and is not entirely emptied till the fourth time.

The mother comes forward. Her hair is unbraided and loose, for the mother's hair is kept loose from the time of the birth of the child until this ceremony, to signify her holiness. When a girl goes through her puberty rite, she has her hair down also. After this ceremony the mother can do her hair in braids again.

The singer cuts four strips of deerskin from an unblemished and

shamans angered them and they burst through the vault of the underworld to this earth. The people followed in order to regain "the light." This passage conveys the Jicarilla conception of ceremonialism as a series of protective devices which carry men safely from one crisis to another until life's end.

4. The sacred substances used and the ritual patterns observed in this rite constitute a good introduction to these phases of Jicarilla ceremonialism.

tanned buck or doeskin, one which has not been shot with an arrow or a bullet and therefore has no holes or cuts in it. He ties the strips together, end to end, making one long strip. He paints it red with red ochre while he sings. He puts pollen and then specular iron ore on it four times from end to end. This string is called "spider's thread." He raises the string and motions with it as though stretching it out. He holds one end to the baby's chest and stretches out the other end, giving the baby long life. He is facing the east all the while. He presses the string against the baby's chest and then against its back. If the child is a boy, he ties a piece of turquoise to one end of the string now; if it is a girl, he uses a piece of abalone. Then he puts the string down on the baby's clothes which have been laid before him.

He starts now to paint the baby's face.[5] He uses the palm of his hand and paints the entire face with red ochre. Then he paints the mother's face, and next the father's. If other children of the mother are present, or any other children or adults, the singer paints them too. After this, pollen is put on the baby's face and on the faces of the others in the same order. Then the same is done with specular iron ore. The man is singing all the time he is doing this.

When all are painted, he motions four times with the baby, and the fourth time hands it to the father saying, "This is your baby."[6] The father receives the baby, motions four times to the mother, and gives the baby to her the fourth time.

At the end of the ceremony the singer ties the string around the baby. He begins at the top of the baby's body and spirals it down along the body. The stone or shell is at the top. This string is kept on the child all the time till he walks around. After that the mother keeps it with the umbilical cord. She is supposed to keep it all her life.

The whole ceremony is over before noon. Its length depends on how many songs the man sings and how he conducts it. After the ceremony, they eat; all the relatives and friends come in the morning and are fed. They don't stay all day, though.

— *Morris Edward Opler*

5. Face painting has the force of a prayer and a blessing in Jicarilla ceremonialism.
6. The social responsibility of the man to his family and, indeed, to his wife's close kin as well, is one of the important aspects of the Jicarilla social system. It is interesting that the husband's obligations to his wife and child are so explicitly and publicly stated.

63: Eskimo Birth Customs

During childbirth old women who are reputed to have skill in such matters act as midwives. Formerly, among the Unalit, when a woman was confined with her first child she was considered unclean and put out in a tent or other shelter by herself for a certain period. This custom is now becoming obsolete, but it is still observed by the Eskimo of Kaviak Peninsula, by the Malamute, and by other remote tribes. In one case that came to my knowledge a young Malamute woman was confined with her first child at a village on the lower Yukon. It was midwinter, but she was put outside in a small brush hut covered with snow and her food handed her by her husband through a small opening. Despite the intensely cold weather, she was kept there for about two months.

When a child is born it is given the name of the last person who died in the village, or the name of a deceased relative who may have lived in another place. The child thus becomes the namesake and representative of the dead person at the feast to the dead, as described under the heading of that festival. In case the child is born away from the village, at a camp or on the tundra, it is commonly given the name of the first object that catches its mother's eyes, such as a bush or other plant, a mountain, a lake, or other natural object.

The name thus given is sometimes changed. When a person becomes old he takes a new name, hoping thereby to obtain an extension of life. The new name given is usually indicative of some personal peculiarity, and, after a person makes a change of this kind, it is considered improper to mention the former one. Some of the Malamute dislike very much to pronounce their own names, and if a man be asked his name he will appear confused and will generally turn to a bystander, asking him to give the desired information.

Formerly it was a common custom to kill female children at birth if they were not wanted, and girls were often killed when from four to six years of age. Children of this sex are looked upon as a burden, since they are not capable of contributing to the food supply of the family, while they add to the number of persons to be maintained. When infants are killed they are taken out naked to the graveyard and there exposed to the cold, their mouths being filled with snow, so that they will freeze to death quickly.

Near St. Michael I saw a young Malamute girl of ten or twelve years, who, soon after birth, had been exposed in this manner with her mouth filled with snow. Fortunately for the child, this occurred close to a trading station. By accident the trader found her a few moments later, and by threats succeeded in making the mother take her back. The child was afterward reared without further attempt on the part of the parents to take its life.

One of the Eskimo told me that if a man had a girl not more than five or six years old who cried much, or if he disliked it for any reason, or found it difficult to obtain food for the family, he would take it far out on the ice at sea or on the tundra during a severe snowstorm, and there abandon it to perish by exposure.

A man at St. Michael was in my house one day and told me in a casual way that his wife had given birth to another girl, and added, "At first I was going to throw it away on the tundra, and then I could not, for it was too dear to me." This man was one of the most intelligent Eskimo I knew. He had been associated with the Russians and other white men since early boyhood, and was one of the so-called converts of the Russian church; yet the idea that a man was not perfectly justified in disposing of a girl child as he saw fit never for a moment occurred to him.

On the other hand, a pair of childless Eskimo frequently adopt a child, either a girl or a boy, preferably the latter. This is done so that when they die there will be someone left whose duty it will be to make the customary feast and offerings to their shades at the festival of the dead. All of the Eskimo appear to have great dread of dying without being assured that their shades will be remembered during the festivals, fearing if neglected that they would thereby suffer destitution in the future life.

In March, 1880, while on a journey to Sledge Island, just south of Bering Strait, we were accompanied for the last seventy-five miles by the wife of our Eskimo interpreter, who was a fine-looking woman of about thirty years and was heavy with child. She went with us in order that her confinement might take place among her own people, who lived on the island. Notwithstanding her condition, she tramped steadily through the snow with the rest of us day after day, and on the morning of our arrival at the island she was in the room with us talking and laughing when she became suddenly ill, went to her mother's house, and was delivered of a fine boy in less than half an hour. Directly after the birth a shaman came in and borrowed from me a drum and a small ivory carving of a white whale, which I had purchased on the road. The father explained that the image of the whale was borrowed to put in the child's mouth so as to feed him upon something that would make him grow up a fine hunter. The shaman beat the drum and sang for half an hour over the boy to make him stouthearted and manly. The woman remained at this village a few days and then walked back the seventy-five miles to her home, carrying the child on her back.

—Edward Wilson Nelson

64: Twinning in Yoruba

Hail,
Twins, worthy to be praised,
Pitifully small
In the eyes of the cowife,
Two infants splendidly alive
In the eyes of their own mother.

The astonishingly high rate of fraternal twins among the Yoruba — forty-two in a total of 117 births in one reliable sample — and the relatively higher degree of infant mortality prevalent in twinning combine to suggest one reason for a prodigious quantity of sculptures for departed twins in Yorubaland, a tradition first noted in writing by the explorer Richard Lander on about 7 April 1830 at the village of Ibeshe:

> Many women with little wooden figures on their heads passed in the course of the morning, mothers who, having lost a child, carry imitations of them about their persons for an indefinite time as a symbol of mourning. None could be induced to part with these affectionate little memorials.

He met twin sculptures again at Pooya, between Ijana and Asunora:

> Whenever the mother stopped to take refreshment, a small part of their food was invariably presented to the lips of these inanimate memorials.

Lander's materials illustrate clearly maternal love of the twins and religious conviction, the latter quality suggested by the feeding of the images as if they were alive, both more convincing motives for the rise of the cult than factors of morbidity per se. High twinning and infant mortality are present in much of Black Africa and yet only in Yoruba and Yoruba-influenced territory is there a tradition of sculpture for the twins. To the immediate west of Yoruba, the Fon and Ewe carve small images in memory of twins; while to the north, the people of Kaiama in Borgu make highly abstract images, called *isabi agba,* which are possibly related to the tradition. These camwood-painted structures resemble ancient stem-on-cone crowns, with rich cowrie fringes adding to the illusion. Remarkable emblems, *isabi agba* hint of riches, in the use of cowrie money as embellishment, and the royalty of the past in the crownlike shape. It is significant that William Fagg collected information to the effect that *isabi agba* are considered the greatest of the ancestors of Kaima and brought wealth to the people and popularity to the kings.

The Borgu vision of inherent riches links the *isabi agba* to a song sung far away in Cuba by descendants of Yoruba slaves:

Beji, beji la
O be ekun iya re

Give birth to twins! And be rich!
Give birth to twins! And be rich!
Twins console their weeping mother.
(She will weep no more from hunger.)

This takes us back, according to Yoruba traditions shared with the writer by the Araba of Lagos, to the foundation of the twin cult, centuries and centuries ago, when only the poor and the wretched were believed to be progenitors of twins, and when the twins were put to death at birth. Then came the day when the children of Oyo people in the region of Ayashe — the modern Porto Novo — began to die mysterious deaths and alarmed parents consulted the oracle. The word of the oracle was clear: cease killing twins at once and honor them to persuade them from killing other children. And it was done. The mothers of the twins began to worship twins every five days, and to dance about, and receive money for their dancing. This made once-poor families relatively rich. Today the mother of twins in traditional areas may dance in a public place where she receives money even if she is of means. Hence the coming of twins is associated with a rise in the fortune of the family and there is rejoicing.

—Robert Farris Thompson

65: Baptism Lore

The time between birth and baptism was especially dangerous, and both mother and child were open to attacks from evil spirits. The child particularly was liable to be stolen by fairies, and a changeling left in its place. To avert these perils, a piece of iron, or some salt, or the father's coat were put on the bedfoot; or the bed itself was "sained" by carrying a lighted torch or candle round it. The protective power of fire and salt against all forms of evil was very great. An unchristened child was sometimes given an egg, a handful of salt and a box of matches — the last being connected with fire and, like the salt, intended as a safeguard. In some places, a pinch of salt was put in the baby's mouth on its first visit to another house. In the North of England, the father's clothes were laid over a girl, and the mother's petticoat over a boy to make the child attractive to the opposite sex.

The folklore of baptism is a curious mixture of Christian and pagan beliefs. The rite itself occurs in many non-Christian religions in places as far apart as Scandinavia and New Zealand. The Druids had a form of baptism; the heathen Norsemen had a naming ceremony with water which was important because the right of inheritance depended on it, and because a child could not afterwards be exposed. Both religion and folklore urge early christening. A child who dies unbaptized is thought to be shut out from heaven, and for this reason it cannot be buried in consecrated ground. In Devon such a child becomes one of the Yeth Hounds who hunt over the moor with the Devil. Butterflies are often said to be the souls of unchristened babies or, in Nidderdale, nightjars. A belief that was formerly widely held was that they joined the hosts of the fairies, who were looked upon as intermediate spirits, not good enough for heaven or bad enough for hell. Witches were often accused of using the fat of unbaptized infants for their spells, and while the ceremony was postponed the child remained in danger of being stolen by them or by fairies.

In the north of England, the graves of stillborn children were carefully avoided, for to step on one might bring on "grave-merels" or "grave-scab," a disease whose symptoms were a trembling of the limbs, difficulty in breathing, and a burning skin. But in the south and west to bury such a child, who was sinless, in an open grave meant that the next person laid in it would be certain of heaven.

—*Christina Hole*

66: Baptism Lore

If a child cries during baptism it is the Devil leaving him. If twins be brought to baptism at the same time, christen the boy first, or else he will have no beard, and the girl will be beggared.

When a child is baptized it is given a few teaspoonsful of baptismal water so that it may be bright and a good singer.

If in baptism the child does not receive the name intended for it, it will not live long.

To decline to act as sponsor at a baptism will bring misfortune.

Wash a child with the water of baptism and it will have a beautiful complexion. Baptism should be done during the full moon to bring good luck.

The last baby to leave the church during a mass baptism is liable to sickness. The sponsors carry the child to the house and kneel before the parents and present the child with a promise that they, too, have the parents' obligations and duties. Then they wash their hands in water and place money in it as a sign of abundance to the child in later life.

— *collected by Fanny D. Bergen, Edwin M. Fogel,*
and Francisco R. Demetrio

67: Welsh Childbirth Lore

There is a Welsh proverb to the effect that a good workman is known in his cradle. If a child in the cradle does not look up at you, it will be deceitful. A child with two crowns to its head will be lucky in money matters. If seven girls are born in succession, the youngest will be a witch or gifted with second sight. If seven boys are born in succession, the youngest will have the power to heal by the passing of his hands over the affected parts. He will also be lucky in planting and sowing, for "everything will grow after him."

Children born with cauls around their heads will be very fortunate, and they will never be drowned. The caul is bought by mariners for their ships. So long as it is on board the vessel will not be shipwrecked. Fastened securely to the figurehead of the ship, it is protection against lightning and disasters by fire or meteoric showers. A child born on a Sunday will be fortunate. If born three hours after sunrise on that day, the child will be able to converse with spirits. Babes born on the last two days of the week are said to marry late in life. When a child suffers from hiccoughs, he is said to be thriving. If two children who cannot talk kiss each other, one will surely die within the year. The first time a child is carried out, one of its garments should be put on with the wrong side uppermost for luck. If a newly born infant cries, three keys should be placed in the bottom of the cradle. If an infant learns to say "Dada" first, the next child will be a boy; if it says "Mam" first, the next child will be a girl.

In the past it was customary for the nurse to place a Prayer Book or a hymn book in the bed until a babe was baptized. A fire was always kept burning in the room where the infant was born. This was done to keep the devil away, and prevent the fairies from changing the child. The

Welsh would never have a child baptized after a funeral, for they said it would thus be prevented from following the dead to the grave during its infancy or early years. They disliked christening a babe on the anniversary of its brother's or sister's birth.

If a babe holds its head up during the christening ceremony, it will live to be very old; if it allows its head to turn aside or sink back on the arm of the person who holds it you may expect its early death.

Christenings never take place on Fridays in Wales. The old people say: "The child that is christened on Friday will grow up to be a rogue."

Whatever a baby first clutches will indicate its future occupation.

While a knife, a ball of yarn, and a key remain in an infant's cradle, it will not be under the influence of sorcery.

A woman who is about to become a mother is not allowed to salt a pig or touch any part of the killed meat, or make butter, or do any kind of dairy work. This is of general occurrence in the present day, for the touch of the woman is regarded as pernicious.

She must not walk or step over a grave. If she does so, her child will have coarse hands. If she ties a cord around her waist, her child will be unlucky. If she turns the washing tubs upside down as soon as she has finished with them, her child will be tidy and orderly. If she passes through any kind of tangle, her child will have a life of confusion. If she meddles much with flowers, her child will not have a keen sense of smell. If she has a great longing for fish, her child will be born too soon, or will soon die. "She must not spin," said people in the eighteenth century; "for if she does, flax or hemp will be made into a rope that will hang her child." If, instead of eating at a table, she goes to the cupboard and "picks at food," her child will be a glutton.

If she dusts her furniture with her apron, her children will be very disorderly.

It is lucky for mother and child if a spinster passes in and out of the room at the time of the birth.

Children should not be weaned at the time when birds migrate to or from Britain. If they are weaned at that period, they become restless and very changeable. If weaned when the trees are in blossom, they will have prematurely grey hair.

Old Welsh nurses would not allow rattles to be given to the children, because they made the latter "late in talking" or "very slow of speech." If you bathe babies in rainwater, they will talk early and be good conversationalists.

If you rock an empty cradle, you will take the infant's rest away.

The first time a baby's nails need paring the mother bites them off. If she cuts them, the child will be a thief.

If you blow the baby's first food to cool it, the child will never be scalded in the mouth.

A horseshoe placed under the pillow of a child subject to convulsions would cure the malady. Children beloved by the fairies died young. When babies smiled or laughed in their sleep, the Welsh nurses in the long-ago said the fairies were kissing them. If a child in the cradle would not look at you, it would be a witch. It was customary to place a small bag of salt in the cradle until the baby was baptized to protect the babe from witches.

To insure good luck for a newly born babe, a pair of tongs or a knife was placed in the cradle the day before the christening. A piece of braid made of the child's mother's hair was used for the same purpose.

The Welsh peasantry believe that children born when the moon is new will be very eloquent. Those born at the last quarter will have excellent reasoning powers. Girls born while the moon is waxing will be precocious.

People formerly said if you wanted your children to attain a long age, you should see that the godparents come from three different parishes. If you stride over a child who is crawling on the floor, you will stop its growth. Newly born babes should not be laid on their left sides first, for they will be awkward in shape and clumsy in movement. If a babe is weaned, and afterwards suckled again, it will become a profane swearer when grown up. If you measure a child for garments in the first six months of its life, it will often want clothes. When a child dies, they say it visits the person who was fondest of it. If a newborn babe is wrapped in fur, its hair will be curly.

A child who has not yet talked should never be held up to a mirror, for this encourages vanity.

A child with small ears will never grow to be rich, while a babe with very large ears will live to be selfish and a great talker. A nearsighted baby will be a saving man. Red birthmarks around the neck of a child are called the "hangman's sign," and he will come to the gallows. If the baby's eyes are beady, he will be untruthful. The old women say: "Watch well when the child has finished cutting its first teeth, for if there is a parting between the two front teeth to admit the passing of a sixpenny piece, that individual will have riches and prosperity all through life." The child who enters the world in an abnormal manner will be gifted with courage, and be able to conquer his enemies. A very precocious child dies early.

It was formerly the custom in Wales to make a large rich cheese for luck, in readiness for the expected birth of the first child. This was made in secret, and not a man was allowed to know of it, especially the husband. When the gossips congregated at the birth, and the husband invited the women to take refreshment, they stolidly refused; but the moment his back was turned out came the cheese and beer! Part of the cheese was eaten, and the remainder was divided among the women, who were expected to take their portions home. All this was done secretly for the sake of good luck and the prosperity of mother and infant.

— *Marie Trevelyan*

68: Tree Planting
at the Birth of a Child

It was formerly a common Jewish custom to plant a tree at the birth of a child, a cedar for a boy, and a pine for a girl. When a couple married, their respective trees were cut down and used in the construction of the *huppah,* or bridal bower.

The custom is mentioned already in the Talmud, but it is probable that the Jews of later generations did not so much inherit it by unbroken tradition as adopt it anew from their Gentile neighbors, for the fact is that, throughout the ages, it has enjoyed widespread popularity in all parts of Europe and Asia. A few examples must suffice.

In Switzerland, it is the practice to plant an apple tree at the birth of a boy, and a nut tree at that of a girl.

In Sweden, an addition to the family is frequently marked by the planting of a tree of destiny (*världträd*) in his or her home.

From Germany comes the familiar story that on the day Goethe was born, his grandfather promptly planted a pear tree in his garden at Frankfort; while a legend from the Aar Valley tells of a father who was so incensed at finding his son a wastrel that he disowned him by cutting down the tree which he had planted at the latter's birth.

Nor, indeed, is the custom unknown in more remote parts of the world. Missionaries have attested to its prevalence in Java, Amboina, Guinea, the Fiji Islands, the Solomons, and New Zealand; while on the Malacca Peninsula there is a special semisacred enclosure in which birth-trees are set up.

The practice is inspired by the idea that the life and destiny of the newborn child are bound up in some mystic fashion with that of the tree. If the latter flourishes, so too will the child, but if it withers or fails to put forth shoots in the season, this is a sure sign that the child faces death or disaster. This idea—itself but one form of what folklorists call the concept of the life-token—is a favorite theme of folktale and legend.

An ancient Egyptian tale relates, for example, that when two brothers parted company, the younger mystically attached his heart to a pine tree, advising the elder that if he should meet with death, the tree would immediately die.

Similarly, in a story from Madagascar, the hero, when setting out on his adventures, plants some *aruns* and plantain trees and informs his parents that "if these wilt, it will be a sign that I am sick; if they wither, that I am dead"; while in the Kalmuk legend of Siddhi Kur, six youths who go forth simultaneously to seek their fortunes each plants a tree the flowering or fading of which will apprise his family how he is faring; and in a Scottish tale from Argyllshire, three trees serve as tokens of the fate and fortune of a fisherman's three sons.

Ancient Roman literature likewise furnishes some arresting instances of this belief. Sabinus, the father of Vespasian, we are told, learned that his newborn son would become a Caesar when he saw an oak tree in his garden suddenly put forth an exceptionally strong branch, and when a laurel sprang up in the house and overshadowed a *malus Persica* or peach tree growing beside it, the father of Alexander Severus was informed by the soothsayers that his son was destined to conquer the Persians.

The motif recurs in the Scandinavian Eddas. Atli is warned that his child has been slain by seeing in a dream that the tree which he had planted at the latter's birth has suddenly become damaged.

Lastly, there is an echo of the idea even in the Bible. For in the Book of Daniel (4:7 ff.), Nebuchadnezzar learns of his impending doom by dreaming nightly of a mighty tree which, though "its height reached to heaven" and though "it could be sighted in every part of the earth," was nevertheless ordered by an angel to be felled.

A variation on the same theme may be recognized in the practice of planting a tree to symbolize the prosperity of a king and the stability of his reign. Such a tree formerly existed in the palace of the Emperor of China; and in Uganda, the life of the sovereign is similarly bound up with that of a tree. Analogous too is the custom observed in the Nile Valley of planting a tree at a wedding to symbolize the future fortune of the bride.

—*Theodor H. Gaster*

69: A Chhohar Mangal Song

After the birth of a child, the Satnami perform a ceremony to ensure its happiness in the world and to give it a name. They sing the following Chhohar Mangal song:

> Where have you come from, little one?
> Where were you staying before?
> Today where have you made your camp?
>
> I came from the sky; till now I was staying in the belly
> Today I have camped on earth.
>
> You came down to the world with your little fists clenched
> You have forgotten the five divine names
> You have forgotten them in love of your new home
> The semur tree climbs up to heaven
> Its cotton flies into the sky and whirls about the world
> Where will it find rest?
>   —*Verrier Elwin*

70: Names and Naming

If a child is christened Eve, she will not live long. There will be no more children in a family after one of them has been named for its mother or father.

It is good luck to have your initials spell a word.

It is bad luck to have thirteen letters in your name.

In esoteric thought, names are an integrating expression of the horoscope. There has been a great deal of speculation about the symbolic elements entering into the composition of names: letters in their graphic or phonetic aspects, similes, analogies, and so on. Piobb, for instance, has suggested that the name Napoleon is Apollo in the Corsican pronunciation of *O'N'Apolio*. The question of why a given name should determine the destiny of one individual but not of another is something which lies beyond the scope of this work. Here we must limit ourselves to describing the rational basis of the symbolism of names and its connection with the Egyptian idea of the "power of words" (as described in a poem by Edgar Allen Poe). Given the symbolic nature of the Egyptian language, it follows that a name could never be a product of change but only of the study of the characteristics of a given thing, whether the name in question was common or proper. The name RN (signifying a mouth over the surface of water) represented the action of the "word" upon passivity. Concerning personal nomenclature, the Egyptians believed that their names were a reflection of their souls. This gave rise to the belief that a name could have a magical effect upon some other person. The equation of a name with character (and destiny) had its repercussions also in descriptive names, such as that of Osiris, which means "he who is at the top of the steps" (the steps, that is, of evolution); or that of Arabia, signifying "he who walks in silence." Onomatopoeia was another highly important source in the genesis of language and its ideographic representation, whereby a given being is characterized by one of its essential aspects—as the lion by its roar, for example: or RW in Egyptian. Popular works on occultism which suggest symbolic implications for certain proper names, as in other cases of vulgarized interpretation, have some roots in authentic symbolism but they may also fall into the trap of being too hard and fast about the true scope of symbolism.

—*Juan Eduardo Cirlot*

71: The Birth-Number

Many numerologists stress the importance of still another number—the Birth-Number—which is found by adding up your date of birth. If you were born on November 14, 1928, for instance, your Birth-Number is 9.

November 14, 1928
$11+14+1+9+2+8=45=4+5=9$

This number is an indication of the stamp which the mysterious forces that move the universe impressed on your character and destiny at the moment you were born. It will affect you all your life and it may not harmonize with the number of your name. If it does not, you can expect to be torn by inner conflict and you may seem to always be struggling against fate.

—Richard Cavendish

72: Childbirth Lore Among
the Chinese

In any Chinese home, whether of the peasantry or the bourgeoisie, the birth of sons and daughters is counted the greatest blessing. They are prayed for (sons especially) in appeals to Sung Tzu Niang Niang who may or may not be considered as a manifestation of Kuan-yin the Goddess of Mercy. Kuan-yin herself is besought for the gift of offspring, especially in cases of childlessness or in danger at childbirth. T'ien Hou is likewise worshipped with similar purpose.

Where childbirth is feared and in cases of special anxiety during pregnancy, sometimes frantic prayers are addressed to T'ai Chün Hsien Niang or Yang T'ai Chün, a goddess of easy childbirths; or it may be that prayers will be offered to Hsieh Jên Hsing Chün, a star-goddess of childbirth, or to Hsieh Kuang Hsing Chün or to T'ien Shêng or Ts'ui Shêng—all in the expectation and express hope of facilitating easy delivery at childbirth.

On the third or seventh day after the birth of a child, the god and goddess of the bed, Ch'uang Kung and Ch'uang P'o are honored with a sacrifice of candies, sweetened rice and sugared wine, after which the child is bathed and bedecked and presented to the household gods and those of the bed in particular. These figures may be pasted on the conjugal bed at weddings, or when a new bed is installed, or at other times, to be implored for good sleep, good health, good disposition for infants, and general peace among the children of the family.

A great protector of children is Chang Hsien the Immortal who is invariably portrayed in the act of shooting his peachwood arrow at the dog in the sky that ravishes children and devours their corpses. As Chang Hsien Sung Tzu, he is constantly invoked for male issue and successful confinement. Another welcome protector of little children is Pao Tung Chiang Chün, the warrior general who has taken this role. To our knowledge there is no grouping of child protectors in Chekiang such as the nine *Niang-Niang* of North China mentioned by Krause and Grube: namely, T'ien Hsien — Heavenly Goddess; Sung Tzu — goddess of child's grace and blessings; Tse-Sun — goddess of posterity; Ts'ui Shêng — goddess of easy childbirth; Nai Mu — goddess of wet nurses; P'ei-Yang — goddess of nourishment; Yen-Kuang — goddess of babies' eyesight; Tou-Chên — goddess of smallpox; and Pan-Chên — goddess of scarlet fever.

Peasant families have recourse also to many *ma-chang* figures which are thought to assist in the rearing of children. Such, for example, is K'ai Kuan Hsing, literally the "Open-Shut Star" whose sole function is to assist children through the peculiarly trying periods of early infancy and adolescence. Special offerings are made to it on the child's hundredth day; as also on its third, sixth, and ninth birthdays. The early education of children is placed in the care of Tzu I who is supposed to guide the studies of young kindergartners.

Birthdays and general anniversaries are counted as eventful days in the family life cycle. The lives and fortunes of the individual members are of real concern to the whole group as it gathers to offer congratulations and join in supplications to the gods for continued blessings. More particularly is sacrifice made to Pên Ming Hsin Chün, the Individual Fate Star in charge of every life, male or female. In some places Pên Ming Hsin Chün is the patron star for males, while Hsi Ch'ih Wang Mu, Royal Mother of the Western Pool, is invoked as patroness of female lives, especially of brides. Her origin and identity is a matter of some conjecture among sinologues, a question into which we need not enter here, other than to note that as Queen of the West she is doubtless the same figure as Hou T'u Kuo Huang the symbolic *Yin,* or Sovereign Earth Goddess who resides in the K'un-lun Mountains of West China. Whether she is to be identified with the Greek goddess Hera, or with the Queen of Sheba, does not concern us here. For the peasant buyers of *ma-changs,* she is the woman's long life protectress, of great power because of great age herself. Her symbol is a peach tree, or in her hand is held the peach of long life. Wang Mu and Pên Ming are especially praised on occasions like the sixtieth birthdays of women or men. Wang Mu is blessed, too, on the arrival of a girl baby, and by one of Hangchow's *ma-chang* sellers she was classed as the greatest of the Pa Hsien, the Eight Immortals whose magic power is a household byword.

—Clarence B. Day

73: On the Birth of His Son

Families, when a child is born
Want it to be intelligent.
I, through intelligence,
Having wrecked my whole life,
Only hope the baby will prove
Ignorant and stupid.
Then he will crown a tranquil life
By becoming a Cabinet Minister.
— *Su Tung-p'o (1036–1101)*

74: Prayer Spoken While Presenting an Infant to the Sun

Now this is the day.
Our child,
Into the daylight
You will go out standing.
Preparing for your day,
We have passed our days.
When all your days were at an end,
When eight days were past,
Our sun father
Went in to sit down at his sacred place.
And our night fathers,
Having come out standing to their sacred place,
Passing a blessed night.
Now this day,
Our fathers, Dawn priests
Have come out standing to their sacred place,
Our sun father,
Having come out standing to his sacred place,
Our child, it is your day.
This day,
The flesh of the white corn, prayer meal,
To our sun father
This prayer meal we offer.

May your road be fulfilled.
Reaching to the road of your sun father.
When your road is fulfilled,
In your thoughts may we live.

May we be the ones whom your thoughts will embrace,
For this, on this day,
To our sun father,
We offer prayer meal.
To this end:
May you help us all to finish our roads.

75: Naming Song

And when they name you great warrior, then will my
   eyes be wet with remembering.
And how shall we name you, little warrior?
See, let us play at naming.
It will not be a name of despisal, for you are my firstborn.
Not as Nawal's son is named will you be named.
Our gods will be kinder to you than theirs.
Must we call you "Insolence" or "Worthless One"?
Shall you be named, like a child of ill fortune, after the dung of cattle?
Our gods need no cheating, my child:
They wish you no ill.
They have washed your body and clothed it with beauty.
They have set a fire in your eyes.
And the little, puckering ridges of your brow—
Are they not the seal of their fingerprints when they fashioned you?
They have given you beauty and strength, child of my heart,
And wisdom is already shining in your eyes, and laughter.

So how shall we name you, little one?
Are you your father's father, or his brother, or yet another?
Whose spirit is that that is in you, little warrior?
Whose spear-hand tightens round my breast?
Who lives in you and quickens to life like last year's melon seeds?
Are you silent, then?
But your eyes are thinking, thinking,
And glowing like the eyes of a leopard in a thicket.
Well, let it be.
At the day of naming you will tell us.

O my child, now indeed I am happy.
Now indeed I am a wife —
No more a bride, but a Mother-of-one.
Be splendid and magnificent, child of desire.
Be proud, as I am proud.
Be happy, as I am happy.
Be loved, as now I am loved.
Child, child, child, love I have had from my man.
But now, only now, have I the fullness of love.
Now, only now, am I his wife and the mother of his firstborn.
His soul is safe in your keeping, my child,
And it was I, I, I, who have made you.
Therefore am I loved.
Therefore am I happy.
Therefore am I a wife.
Therefore have I great honor.

You will tend his shrine when he is gone.
With sacrifice and oblation you will recall his name year by year.
He will live in your prayers, my child,
And there will be no more death for him,
But everlasting life springing from your loins.

You are his shield and spear, his hope and redemption from the dead.
Through you he will be reborn, as the saplings in the Spring.
And I, I am the mother of his first-born.
Sleep, child of beauty and courage and fulfillment, sleep.
I am content.

76: Caul

In folklore, the caul or "veil" is part of the amnion which, for any of several reasons, remains attached to the child when it is born. This is distinctly an omen of good luck, and has been so considered since at least the time of the Romans. The caul, preserved as a talisman, is a protection against drowning. The French proverbial expression "être ne coiffé" is used to characterize those having persistent good fortune. The possessor of a caul obtains from it several magical and medicinal virtues. He can see ghosts and talk to them; even if deaf, he can hear the spirits talk. The caul itself is an amulet partaking of the ideas of the genius and life token. Among the Negroes of Louisiana, it is believed that the owner dies if the caul is torn. As a corollary, a limp caul indicates that the owner is ill, while a firm, crisp caul means that he is in good health. Another American Negro belief, adopted from the English, is that the person born with a caul can tell fortunes. The caul itself is a magic instrument quite apart from its connection with the original possessor. It is widely believed to be a protection against demons, particularly (in Jewish tradition) against storm demons. Hence, the caul is among sailors a valuable protection against drowning. Cauls could be and were sold for high prices.

—Maria Leach

77: Copperfield's Caul

To begin my life with the beginning of my life, I record that I was born on a Friday, at twelve o'clock at night. It was rumored that the clock began to strike, and I began to cry, simultaneously.

In consideration of the day and hour of my birth, it was declared by the nurse, and by some single women in the neighborhood who had taken a lively interest in me several months before there was any possibility of our becoming personally acquainted, first, that I was destined to be unlucky in life, and secondly, that I was privileged to see ghosts and spirits; both these gifts inevitably attaching, as they believed, to all unlucky infants, of either gender, born towards the small hours on a Friday night.

... I was born with a caul, which was advertised for sale in the newspapers, at the low price of fifteen guineas. Whether seagoing peoples were short of money about that time, or were short of faith and preferred cork jackets, I don't know; all I know, is, that there was but one solitary bidding, and that was from an attorney, connected with bill-broking business, who offered two pounds in cash and the balance in sherry, but declined to be guaranteed from drowning on any higher bargain. Consequently, the advertisement was withdrawn at a dead loss—for as to sherry, my poor dear mother's own sherry was in the market then—and ten years afterwards the caul was put up in a raffle down in our part of the county, to fifty members at half a crown a head, the winner to spend five shillings. I was present myself, and remember to have felt quite uncomfortable and confused at a part of myself being disposed of in that way.

—Charles Dickens

78: Prayer of a Mother Whose Child Died

When it is the first-born child of the one who has just for the first time given birth, a young woman, then the woman is really fond of her child. Then she engages a carver to make a little canoe and all kinds of playthings for the boy. And if it is a girl, then she engages a doll maker to make dolls of alder wood, and women are hired by her to make little mats and little dishes and little spoons. Then her child begins to get sick, and not long is sick the child when it dies and the woman carries in her arms her child. Then all the relatives of the woman come to see her and all the women wail together. As soon as all the women stop crying the mother of the child speaks aloud. She says:

"Ah, ah, ah! What is the reason, child, that you have done this to me? I have tried hard to treat you well when you came to me to have me for your mother. Look at all your toys. What is the reason that you desert me, child? May it be that I did something, child, to you in the way I treated you, child? I will try better when you come back to me, child. Please, only become at once well in the place to which you are going. As soon as you are made well, please, come back to me, child. Please, do not stay away there. Please, only have mercy on me who is your mother, child," says she.

Then they put the child in the coffin, and they put it up on a hemlock tree. That is the end.

—*Franz Boas*

79: On the Death of a New Born Child

The flowers in bud on the trees
Are pure like this dead child.
The east wind will not let them last.
It will blow them into blossom,
And at last into the earth.

It is the same with this beautiful life
Which was so dear to me.
While his mother is weeping tears of blood,
Her breasts are still filling with milk.
    — Mei Yao Ch'en (1002–1060)

80: Skip-Rope Rhyme

Fudge, fudge, tell the judge.
Mother had a newborn baby.
It isn't a girl and it isn't a boy,
It's just a fair young lady.
Wrap it up in tissue paper
And send it up the elevator.
First floor, miss.
Second floor, miss.
Fourth floor.
Kick it out the elevator door!
(Player jumps out of the circle . . .)

81: Sung by a Little Girl
to Soothe a Crying Baby

Do not weep, little one,
Your mother will fetch you,
Mother is coming for you
As soon as she has finished
Her new kamiks.

Do not weep, little one,
Your father will fetch you,
Father is coming as soon as he has made
His new harpoon head,
Do not weep, little one,
        Do not weep!

82: Lullaby

Blue-eyed beauty,
Do your mammy's duty;
Black-eye, pick a pie,
Run around and tell a lie;
Gray-eye, greedy gut,
Eat the whole world up.

83: Lullaby

I would put my own child to sleep,
And not the same as the wives of the clowns do,
Under a yellow blanket and a sheet of tow,
But in a cradle of gold rocked by the mind.
　Sho-heen sho, hoo lo lo,
　Sho-heen sho, you are my child,
　Sho-heen sho, hoo lo lo,
　Sho-heen sho, and you are my child.

I would put my own child to sleep,
On the fine sunny day between two Christmases,
In a cradle of gold on a level floor,
Under the tops of boughs and rocked by the wind,
　Sho-heen sho, hoo lo lo, etc.

Sleep, my child, and be it the sleep of safety,
And out of your sleep may you rise in health;
May neither colic nor death-stitch strike you,
The infant's disease, or the ugly smallpox.
　Sho-heen sho, hoo lo lo, etc.

Sleep, my child, and be it the sleep of safety,
And out of your sleep may you rise in health;
From painful dreams may your heart be free,
And may your mother be not a sonless woman.
　Sho-heen sho, hoo lo lo, etc.

84: Lullaby

Ro-ro-ro
Child, why are you crying?
Child, is it for the fat of the monitor lizard?
Give the whole of it.
Child, why are you crying?
Child, is it for the gonala yams you are crying?
Give all of them.
Child, why are you crying?
Child, is it for the head of the wandura monkey?
Give the whole of it.
Child, why are you crying?
Child, is it for the head of the rilawa monkey?
Give the whole of it.
Ro-ro-ro.
Child, creeping child;
are you crying for sleep?
Ro-ro-ro
Darling, Ro-ro-ro.
Darling, for what are you crying?
Darling, is it for bathing you are crying?
Child, what are you crying for?
Child, is it for sleep?
Darling, Ro-ro-ro.

85: Child and Its Synonyms

Our word *child*—the good old English term; for both *babe* and *infant* are borrowed—simply means the "product of the womb" (compare Gothic *kilthei*, "womb"). The Lowland-Scotch dialect still preserves an old word for "child" in *bairn*, cognate with Anglo-Saxon *bearn*, Icelandic, Swedish, Danish, and Gothic *barn* (the Gothic had a diminutive *barnilo*, "baby"), Sanskrit *bharna*, which signifies "the borne one," "that which is born," from the primitive Indo-European root *bhr*, "to bear, to carry in the womb," whence our "to *bear*" and the German "*gebären*." *Son*, which finds its cognates in all the principal Aryan dialects, except Latin, and perhaps Celtic—the Greek υἱός is for συιος, and is the same word—a widespread term for "male child, or descendant," originally meant, as the Old Irish *suth*, "birth, fruit," and the Sanskrit *sû*, "to bear, to give birth to," indicate, "the fruit of the womb, the begotten"—an expression which meets us time and again in the pages of the Hebrew Bible. The words *offspring, issue, seed,* used in higher diction, explain themselves and find analogues all over the world. To a like category belong Sanskrit *gárbha*, "brood of birds, child, shoot"; Pali *gabbha*, "womb, embryo, child"; Old High German *chilburra*, "female lamb"; Gothic *kalbô*, "female lamb one year old"; German *Kalb*; English *calf*; Greek δελφύς, "womb"; whence ἀδελφός, "brother," literally "born of the same womb." Here we see, in the words for their young, the idea of the kinship of men and animals in which the primitive races believed. The "brought forth" or "born" is also the signification of the Niskwalli Indian *ba'-ba-ad*, "infant"; *de-bād-da*, "infant, son"; Maya *al*, "son or daughter of a woman"; Cakehiquel λahol, "son," and like terms in many other tongues. Both the words in our language employed to denote the child before birth are borrowed. *Embryo*, with its cognates in the modern tongues of Europe, comes from the Greek ἔμβρυον, "the fruit of the womb before delivery; birth; the embryo, foetus; a lamb newly born, a kid." The word is derived from ἐν, "within"; and βρύω, "I am full of anything, I swell or teem with"; in a transitive sense, "I break forth." The radical idea is clearly "swelling," and cognates are found in Greek βρύον, "moss"; and German *Kraut*, "plant, vegetable." *Foetus* comes to us from Latin, where it meant "a bearing, offspring, fruit; bearing, dropping, hatching—of animals, plants, etc.; fruit, produce, offspring, progeny, brood." The immediate derivation of the word is from *fētō*, "I breed," whence also *effētus*, "having brought forth young, worn out by bearing, effete." *Fētō* itself is from an old verb *feuere*, "to generate, to produce," possibly related to *fui* and our *be*. The radical signification of *foetus* then is "that which is bred, or brought to be"; and from the same root *fē* are derived *fēles*, "cat" (the fruitful animal); *fē-num*, "hay"; *fē-cundus*, "fertile"; *fē-lix*, "happy" (fruitful). The corresponding verb in Greek is φύειν, "to grow, to spring forth, to come into being," whence the following: φύσις, "a creature, birth, nature"—nature is "all that has had birth"; φυτόν, "something grown, plant, tree, creature, child"; φϋλή, φῖλον, "race, clan, tribe"—the "aggregate of those born in a certain way or place"; φύς, "son"; φύσας, "father," etc.

In English, we formerly had the phrase "to look *babies* in the eyes," and we still speak of the *pupil* of the eye, the old folk-belief having been able to assert itself in the everyday speech of the race—the thought that the soul looked out of the windows of the eyes. In Latin, *pūpilla pūpila*, "girl, pupil of the eye," is a diminutive of *pūpa* (*puppa*), "girl, damsel, doll, puppet"; other related words are *pūpulus*, "little boy"; *pūpillus*, "orphan, ward," our *pupil*; *pūpulus*, "little child, boy"; *pūpus*, "child, boy." The radical of all these is *pu*, "to beget"; whence are derived also the following: *pŭer*, "child, boy"; *pŭella* (for *puerula*), a diminutive of *puer*, "girl"; *pūsus*, "boy"; *pūsio* "little boy"; *pŭsillus*, "a very little boy"; *pŭtus*, "boy"; *pŭtillus*, "little boy"; *pŭtilla*, "little girl"—here belongs also *pusillanimus*, "small-minded, boy-minded"; *pūbis*, "ripe, adult"; *pūbertas*, "puberty, maturity"; *pullus*, "a young animal, a fowl," whence our *pullet*. In Greek we find the cognate words πῶλος, "a young animal," related to our *foal, filly*; πωλιόν, "pony," and, as some, perhaps too venturesome, have suggested, παῖς, "child," with its numerous derivatives in the scientific nomenclature and phraseology of today. In Sanskrit we have *putra*, "son," a word familiar as a suffix in river names—*Brahmaputra*, "son of Brahma"—*pota*, "the young of an animal," etc. Skeat thinks that our word *boy*, borrowed from Low German and probably related to the Modern High German *Bube*, whence the familiar "bub" of American colloquial speech, is cognate with Latin *pūpus*.

227

To this stock of words our *babe,* with its diminutive *baby,* seems not akin. Skeat, rejecting the theory that it is a reduplicative child-word, like *papa,* sees in it merely a modification (infantine, perhaps) of the Celtic *maban,* diminutive of *mab,* "son," and hence related to *maid,* the particular etymology of which is discussed elsewhere.

Infant, also, is a loan word in English. In Latin, *infans* was the coinage of some primitive student of children, of some prehistoric anthropologist, who had a clear conception of "infancy" as "the period of inability to speak," for *infans* signifies neither more nor less than "not speaking, unable to speak." The word, like our "childish," assumed also the meanings "child, young, fresh, new, silly," with a diminutive *infantulus.* The Latin word *infans* has its representatives in French and other Romance languages, and has given rise to *enfanter,* "to give birth to a child," *enfantement,* "labor," two of the few words relating to childbirth in which the child is directly remembered. The history of the words *infantry,* "footsoldiers," and *Infanta,* "a princess of the blood royal" in Spain (even though she be married), illustrates a curious development of thought.

Our word *daughter,* which finds cognates in Teutonic, Slavonic, Armenian, Zend, Sanskrit, and Greek, Skeat would derive from the root *dugh,* "to milk," the "daughter" being primitively the "milker"—the "milkmaid"—which would remove the term from the list of names for "child" in the proper sense of the word. Kluge, however, with justice perhaps, considers this etymology improbable.

A familiar phrase in English is "babes and sucklings," the last term of which, cognate with German *Säugling,* meets with analogues far and wide among the peoples of the earth. The Latin words for children in relation to their parents are *filius* (diminutive *filiolus*), "son," and *filia* (diminutive *filiola*), "daughter," which have a long list of descendants in the modern Neo-Latin or Romance languages, French *fils, fille, filleul,* etc.; Italian *figlio, figlia,* etc. According to Skeat, *filius* signified originally "infant," perhaps "suckling," from *fēlare,* "to suck," the radical of which, *fē* (Indo-European *dhē*), appears also in *fēmina,* "woman," and *fěmella,* "female," the "sucklers" *par excellence.* In Greek the cognate words are τίτθη, "nurse," θῆλυς, "female," θηλή, "teat," etc.; in Lithuanian, *dēls,* "son." With *nonagan,* "teat, breast," are cognate in the Delaware Indian language *nonoshellaan,* "to suckle," *nonetschik,* "suckling," and other primitive tongues have similar series.

The Modern High German word for child is *Kind,* which, as a substantive, finds representatives neither in Gothic nor in early English, but has cognates in the Old Norse *kunde,* "son," Gothic *-kunds,* Anglo-

Saxon -*kund*, a suffix signifying "coming from, originating from." The ultimate radical of the word is the Indo-European root *gen* (Teutonic *ken*), "to bear, to produce," whence have proceeded also *kin*, Gothic *kuni*; *queen*, Gothic *qvêns*, "woman"; *king*, Modern High German *König*, originally signifying perhaps "one of high origin"; Greek γίνος and its derivatives; Latin *genus, gens, gigno*; Lithuanian *gentis*, "relative"; Sanskrit *janas*, "kin, stock," *janús*, "creature, kin, birth," *jantú*, "child, being, stock," *jâlá*, "son." *Kind*, therefore, while not the same word as our *child*, has the same primitive meaning, "the produced one," and finds further cognates in *kid* and *colt*, names applied to the young of certain animals, and the first of which, in the slang of today, is applied to children also. In some parts of Germany and Switzerland *Kind* has the sense of *boy*; in Thuringia, for example, people speak of *zwei Kinder und ein Mädchen*, "two boys and a girl." From the same radical sprang the Modern High German *Knabe*, Old High German *chnabo*, "boy, youth, young fellow, servant," and its cognates, including our English *knave*, with its changed meaning, and possibly also German *Knecht* and English *knight*, of somewhat similar import originally.

To the same original source we trace back Greek γενέτηρ, Latin *genitor*, "parent," and their cognates, in all of which the idea of *genesis* is prominent. Here belong, in Greek: γένεσις, "origin, birth, beginning"; γυνή, "woman"; γενεά, "family, race"; γείνομαι, "I beget, produce, bring forth, am born"; γίγνομαι, "I come into a new state of being, become, am born." In Latin: *gigno*, "I beget, bring forth"; *gens*, "clan, race, nation"—those born in a certain way; *ingens*, "vast, huge, great"— "not *gens*," i.e., "born beyond or out of its kind"; *gentilis*, "belonging to the same clan, race, tribe, nation," then, with various turns of meaning, "national, foreign," whence our *gentile, genteel, gentle, gentry*, etc.; *genus*, "birth, race, sort, kind"; *ingenium*, "innate quality, natural disposition"; *ingeniosus*, "of good natural abilities, born well-endowed," hence *ingenious*; *ingenuus*, "native, free-born, worthy of a free man," hence "frank, *ingenuous*"; *progenies*, "descent, descendants, offspring, progeny"; *gener*, "son-in-law"; *genius*, "innate superior nature, tutelary deity, the god born to a place," hence the *genius*, who is "born," not "made"; *genuinus*, "innate, born-in, *genuine*"; *indigena*, "native, born there, *indigenous*"; *generosus*, "of high, noble birth," hence "noble-minded, *generous*"; *genero*, "I beget, produce, engender, create, procreate," and its derivatives *degenero, regenero*, etc., with the many words springing from them. From the same radical *gen* comes the Latin *(g)nascor*, "I am born," whose stem *(g)na* is seen also in *natio*, "the collection of those born," or "the birth," and *natura*, "the world of birth"—like Greek φύσις—for "nations" and "nature" have both "sprung into being." The Latin *germen* (our *germ*), which signified "sprig, offshoot, young bud, sprout, fruit, embryo," probably meant originally simply "growth," from the root *ker*, "to make to grow." From the same Indo-European radical have come the Latin *creare*, "to create, make, produce," with its derivatives *procreare* and *creator*, which we now apply to the Supreme Being, as the "maker" or "producer" of all things. Akin are also *crescere*, "to come forth, to arise, to appear, to increase, to grow, to spring, to be born," and *Ceres*, the name of the goddess of agriculture (growth and creation), whence our word *cereal*; and in Greek Κρόνος, the son of Uranus (Heaven) and Gaea (Earth), κράτος, "strength," and its derivatives ("democracy," etc.).

Another interesting Latin word is *pario*, "I bring forth, produce," whence *parens*, "producer, parent," *partus*, "birth, bearing, bringing forth; young, offspring, foetus, embryo of any creature," *parturio*, *parturitio*, etc. *Pario* is used alike of human beings, animals, birds, fish, while *parturio* is applied to women and animals, and, by Virgil, even to trees—*parturit arbos*, "the tree is budding forth"—and by other writers to objects even less animate.

In the Latin *ēnītor*, "I bring forth or bear children or young"—properly, "I struggle, strive, make efforts"—we meet with the idea of "labor," now so commonly associated with childbearing, and deriving from the old comparison of the tillage of the soil and the bearing of the young. This association existed in Hebrew also, and Cain, the first-born of Adam, was the first agriculturist. We still say the tree *bears* fruit, the land *bears* crops, is *fertile,* and the most characteristic word in English belonging to the category in question is "to *bear*" children, cognate with Modern High German *ge-bären*, Gothic *gabairan*, Latin *ferre* (whence *fertilis*), Greek φέρειν, Sanskrit *bhri*, etc., all from the Indo-European root *bher*, "to carry"—compare the use of *tragen* in Modern High German: *sie trägt ein Kind unter dem Herzen*. The passive verb is "to be born," literally, "to be borne, to be carried, produced," and the noun corresponding, *birth*, cognate with German *Geburt*, and Old Norse *burthr*, which meant "embryo" as well. Related ideas are seen in *burden*, and in the Latin, *fors, fortuna*, for "fortune" is but that which is "borne" or "produced, brought forth," just as the Modern High German *Heil*, "fortune, luck," is probably connected with the Indo-European radical *gen*, "to produce."

Corresponding to the Latin *parentes*, in meaning, we have the Gothic *berusjōs*, "the bearers," or "parents"; we still use in English, "forebears," in the sense of ancestors. The good old English phrase "with child," which finds its analogues in many other languages, has, through false modesty, been almost driven out of literature, as it has been out of conversational language, by *pregnant,* which comes to us from the Latins, who also used *gravidus* — a word we now apply only to animals, especially dogs and ants — and *enceinte,* borrowed from French, and referring to the ancient custom of girding a woman who was with child. Similarly barren of direct reference to the child are *accouchement,* which we have borrowed from French, and the German *Entbindung.*

In German, Grimm enumerates, among other phrases relating to childbirth, the following, the particular meanings and uses of which are explained in his great dictionary: *Schwanger, gross zum Kinde, zum Kinde gehen, zum Kinde arbeiten, ums Kind kommen, mit Kinde, ein Kind tragen, Kindesgross, Kindes schwer, Kinder haben, Kinder bekommen, Kinder kriegen, niederkommen, entbinden,* and the quaint and beautiful *eines Kindes genesen* — all used of the mother. Applied to both parents we find *Kinder machen, Kinder bekommen* (now used more of the mother), *Kinder erzeugen* (more recently, of the father only), *Kinder erzielen.*

Our English word *girl* is really a diminutive (from a stem *gir,* seen in Old Low German *gör,* "a child") from some Low German dialect, and, though it now signifies only "a female child, a young woman," in Middle English *gerl* (*girl, gurl*) was applied to a young person of either sex. In the Swiss dialects today *gurre,* or *gurrli,* is a name given to a "girl" in a depreciatory sense, like our own "girl-boy." In many primitive tongues there do not appear to be special words for "son" and "daughter," or for "boy" and "girl," as distinguished from each other, these terms being rendered "male-child (man-child)," and "female-child (woman-child)" respectively. The "man-child" of the King James version of the Scriptures belongs in this category. In not a few languages, the words for "son" and "daughter" and for "boy" and "girl" mean really "little man" and "little woman" — a survival of which thought meets us in the "little man" with which his elders are even now wont to denominate "the small boy." In the Nahuatl language of Mexico, "woman" is *ciuatl,* "girl" *ciuatontli;* in the Niskwalli, of the state of Washington, "man" is *stobsh,* "boy" *stótomish,* "woman" *sláne,* "girl" *cháchas* (i.e., "small") *sláne;* in the Tacana, of South America, "man" is *dreja,* "boy" *drejave,* "woman" *epuna,* "girl" *epunave.* And but too often the "boys" and "girls" even as mere children are "little men and women" in more respects than that of name.

In some languages the words for "son," "boy," "girl" are from the same root. Thus, in the Mazatec language of Mexico, we find *indidi* "boy," *tzadi* "girl," *indi* "son," and in the Cholona, of Peru, *nun-pullup* "boy," *ila-pullup* "girl," *pul* "son" —where *ila* means "female," and *nun* "male."

In some others, as was the case with the Latin *puella*, from *puer*, the word for "girl" seems derived from that for "boy." Thus, we have in Maya, *mehen* "son," *ix-mehen* "daughter" — *ix-* is a feminine prefix; and in the Jívaro, of Ecuador, *vila* "son," *vilalu* "daughter."

Among very many primitive peoples, the words for "babe, infant, child," signify really "small," "little one," like the Latin *parvus*, the Scotch *wean* (for *wee ane*, "wee one"), etc. In Hawaiian, for example, the "child" is called *keiki*, "the little one," and in certain Indian languages of the Western Pacific slope, the Wiyot *kusha'ma* "child," Yuke *únsil* "infant," Wintun *cru-tut* "infant," Niskwalli *chá chesh* "child (boy)," all signify literally "small," "little one."

Some languages, again, have diminutives of the word for "child," often formed by reduplication, like the *wee wean* of Lowland Scotch, and the *pilpil*, "infant" of the Nahuatl of Mexico.

In the Snanaimuq language, of Vancouver Island, the words *k·ä'ela*, "male infant," and *k·ä'k·ela*, "female infant," mean simply "the weak one." In the Modoc, of Oregon, a "baby" is literally, "what is carried on one's self." In the Tsimshian, of British Columbia, the word *wok·ä'ūts*, "female infant," signifies really "without labrets," indicating that the creature is yet too young for the lip ornaments. In Latin, *liberi*, one of the words for "children," shows on its face that it meant only "children, as opposed to the slaves of the house, *servi*"; for *liberi* really denotes "the free ones." In "the Galibi language of Brazil, *tigami* signifies 'young brother, son, and little child,' indiscriminately."

—*Alexander Francis Chamberlin*

86: A Mother Praises Her Baby

You son of a clear-eyed mother,
You far-sighted one,
How you will see game one day,
You, who have strong arms and legs,
You strong-limbed one,
How surely you will shoot, plunder the Herreros,
And bring your mother their fat cattle to eat,
You child of a strong-thighed father,
How you will subdue strong oxen between your thighs one day,
You who have a mighty penis,
How many and what mighty children you will beget!

Sources

The numbers of the selections in the text correspond to the entry numbers here, so that the sources can be easily identified. Where a given source is used for more than one selection, the later note will refer you back to the original, complete note.
                                                                    D.M.

Introduction: Frobenius, Leo. *Der Kopf als Schicksal*. Munich: K. Wolff, 1924.

Section I heading: Trask, Willard R., translator and editor. *The Unwritten Song: Poetry of the Primitive and Traditional Peoples of the World*. Volume I. NY: The Macmillan Company, 1966.
  1: de Civrieux, Marc. *Watunna: An Orinoco Creation Cycle* (translated and edited by David Guss). Berkeley: North Point Press, 1980.
  2: Feldman, Susan, ed. *African Myths and Tales*. NY: Dell Publishing Company, Inc., 1963.
  3: Robinson, Roland. *Aboriginal Myths and Legends*. Melbourne: Sun Books, 1966.
  4: Ginzberg, Louis. *The Legends of the Jews*. Philadelphia: The Jewish Publication Society of America, 1910. Volume II.
  5: Hall, Manly Palmer. *Man: Grand Symbol of the Mysteries*. Los Angeles: The Philosophical Research Society, Inc., 1947. 5th Edition.
  6: Conze, Edward, translator and editor. *Buddhist Scriptures*. Baltimore: Penguin Books, 1959.
  7: Pritchard, James B., editor. *Ancient Near Eastern Texts Relating to the Old Testament*. Princeton: Princeton University Press, 1955. 2nd Edition.
  8: Farmer, Philip José. *Tarzan Alive: A Definitive Biography of Lord Greystoke*. Garden City: Doubleday and Company, Inc., 1972.
  9: Philostratus. *The Life of Apollonius of Tyana* (translated by F. C. Conybeare). Cambridge: Harvard University Press (Loeb Classical Library), 1912.
 10: Chamberlin, Alexander Francis. *The Child and Childhood in Folk-Thought*. NY: Macmillan and Company, Inc., 1896.
 11: Editor's reworking.
 12: Taylor, Rev. Richard. *Te Ika a Maui; or, New Zealand and its Inhabitants*. London: No publisher listed, 1855.

Section II heading: Freeman, Kathleen, editor and translator. *Ancilla to the Pre-Socratic Philosophers: A Complete Translation of the Fragments in Diels, Fragmente der Vorsokratiker.* Cambridge: Harvard University Press, 1957.

13: Forbes, Thomas Rogers. *The Midwife and the Witch.* New Haven: Yale University Press, 1966.

14: Ginzberg. *The Legends of the Jews.* Volume II. (See number 4.)

15: Pritchard. *Ancient Near Eastern Texts Relating to the Old Testament.* (See number 7.)

16: Chamberlain, Basil H. "Ainu Folk-Tales." In *Folk-Lore Society.* London: Folk-Lore Society Publications, 1888.

17: Evans-Wentz, W. Y., editor and translator. *The Tibetan Book of the Dead or the After-Death Experiences on the Bardo Plane.* NY: Oxford University Press, 1960.

18: Stevenson, Matilda C. "The Zuñi." In *Annual Report of the Bureau of American Ethnology, 1901–02.* Washington, D.C.: Government Printing Office, 1904.

19: Brasch, R. *How Did It Begin? Customs and Superstitions and Their Romantic Origins.* NY: David McKay Company, 1967.

20: Griaule, Marcel. *Conversations with Ogotemmêli: An Introduction to Dogon Religious Ideas* (translated by Daryll Forde). NY: Oxford University Press, 1965.

Section III heading: Budge, E. A. Wallis. *Amulets and Talismans.* New Hyde Park: University Books, 1961.

21: Elwin, Verrier, translator and editor. *Folk Songs of Chattisgarh.* London: Oxford University Press, 1946.

22: Pritchard. *Ancient Near Eastern Texts Relating to the Old Testament.* (See number 7.)

23: Chamberlin. *The Child and Childhood in Folk-Thought.* (See number 10.)

24: Seyffert, Oskar. *A Dictionary of Classical Antiquities: Mythology, Religion, Literature and Art.* (Revised and edited by Henry Nettleship and J. E. Sandys.) London: W. Glaisher Ltd., 1894.

25: Herskovits, Melville J. *Life in a Haitian Valley.* NY: Alfred A. Knopf, Inc., 1937.

26: Gaster, Moses. "Two Thousand Years of a Charm Against the Child-Stealing Witch." In *Folklore,* Volume II, Number 2, June, 1900. London.

27: Mooney, James R. "Sacred Formulas of the Cherokees." In *Annual Review of the Bureau of American Ethnology: 1885–1886.* Washington, D.C.: Government Printing Office, 1891.

28: Forbes. *The Midwife and the Witch.* (See number 13.)

29: Gonzales-Wippler, Migene. *Santería: African Magic in Latin America.* NY: Julian Press, Inc., 1973.

30: Jastrow, Morris. "Babylonian-Assyrian Birth-Omens." In *Religionsgeschichtliche Versuche u. Vorarbeiten;* Volume XIV, Number 5. Selected from various passages by the editor.

31: de Civrieux. *Watunna: An Orinoco Creation Cycle.* (See number 1.)

32: Gifford, Edward S. *The Evil Eye: Studies in the Folklore of Vision.* NY: The Macmillan Company, 1958.

33: Forbes. *The Midwife and the Witch.* (See number 13.)

34: Ibid.

35: Gaster, Theodor H. *The Holy and the Profane.* NY: William Sloane Associates, 1955.

36: Moore, A. W. *The Folk-Lore of the Isle of Man.* London: D. Nutt, 1891.

37: Randolph, Vance. *Ozark Superstitions.* NY: Columbia University Press, 1947.

Browne, Ray B. "Popular Beliefs and Practices from Alabama." In *Folklore Studies: 9.* Berkeley: University of California Press, 1958.

Newman, Lucile F. "Folklore of Pregnancy: Wives' Tales in Contra Costa County, California." In *Western Folklore,* Volume 28, Number 23, 1969. Berkeley: University of California Press.

Bergen, Fanny D., editor. *Current Superstitions from the Oral Tradition of English Speaking Folk.* Boston: Houghton Mifflin and Company, Inc., 1896.

Fogel, Edwin Miller. *Beliefs and Superstitions of the Pennsylvania Germans.* Philadelphia: Americana Germanica Press, 1915.

Hyatt, Harry Middleton. *Folk-Lore from Adams County, Illinois.* NY: The Alma Egan Hyatt Foundation, 1935.

Section IV heading: Ingalls, Daniel H. H., editor and translator. *Sanskrit Poetry from Vidyakara's "Treasury."* Cambridge: Harvard University Press, 1968.

38: Neumann, Erich. *The Great Mother: An Analysis of the Archetype* (translated from the German by Ralph Manheim). NY: Pantheon Books (Bollingen Series XLVII), 1955.

39: Elwin. *Folk Songs of Chattisgarh.* (See number 21.)

40: Diner, Helen. *Mothers and Amazons: The First Feminine History of Culture* (1938) (translated from the German by John Philip Lundlin). NY: Julian Press, Inc., 1965.

41: Chang, Garma C. C., translator and editor. *The Hundred Thousand Songs of Milarepa; The Life-Story and Teaching of the Greatest Poet-Saint Ever to Appear in the History of Buddhism.* New Hyde Park: University Books, 1962. Volume II.

42: Lore collected by the editor.

43: Elwin. *Folk Songs of Chattisgarh.* (See number 21.)

44: Parsons, Elsie Clews. *The Old-Fashioned Woman: Primitive Fancies About the Sex.* NY: G. P. Putnam's Sons, 1913.

Section V heading: Trask. *The Unwritten Song.* Volume I. (See Section I heading.)

45: Opler, Morris Edward. "Childhood and Youth in Jicarilla Apache Society." In *Publications of the Frederick Webb Hodge Society Publication Fund.* Volume 5. Los Angeles: The Southwest Museum/Administrator of the Fund, 1946.

46: Herskovits. *Life in a Haitian Valley.* (See number 25.)

47: Hanks, Jane Richardson. *Maternity and its Rituals in Bang Chan.* (Data Paper #51 of the Southeast Asia Program.) Ithaca: Department of Asian Studies, Cornell University, 1963..

48: King-Hall, Magdalen. *The Story of the Nursery.* London: Routledge and Kegan Paul, 1967.

49: Pukui, Mary Kawena. "Hawaiian Beliefs and Customs During Birth, Infancy, and Childhood." In *Occasional Papers of the Bernice P. Bishop Museum.* Volume 16, Number 17 (March 20, 1942). Honolulu: Bishop Museum Press.

50: Braude, Morris. *Life Begins: Childbirth in Lore and its Literature.* Chicago: Argus Books, 1935.

51: Hanks. *Maternity and its Rituals in Bang Chan.* (See number 47.)

52: Stimson, J. Frank. *Songs and Tales of the Sea Kings: Interpretations of the Oral Literature of Polynesia.* Salem: The Peabody Museum, 1957.

53: Smith, Mary. *Baba of Karo: A Woman of the Moslem Hausa.* NY: Frederick A. Praeger, Publishers, 1964.

54: Redesdale, Lord. *Tales of Old Japan.* London: Macmillan and Company, Ltd., 1906.

55: Stevenson, Matilda C. "The Zuñi." (See number 18.)

56: Fodor, Nandor. *The Search for the Beloved: A Clinical Investigation of the Trauma of Birth and Pre-Natal Condition.* New Hyde Park: University Books, Inc., 1949.

57: Cendrars, Blaise. "My Mother's Womb." Translated from the French by Denis Kelly.

58: Elwin. *Folk Songs of Chattisgarh.* (See number 21.)

59: Forbes. *The Midwife and the Witch.* (See number 13.)

60: Feldman. *African Myths and Tales.* (See number 2.)

61: Rombandeeva, E. I. "Some Observations and Customs of the Mansi (Voguls) in Connection with Childbirth." In *Popular Beliefs and Folklore Traditions in Siberia,* edited by V. Dioszegi. Bloomington: Indiana University (The Uralic and Altaic Series), 1960.

Section VI heading: Blake, William. "Infant Joy." (The definitive collection of Blake's poems is *The Poetry and Prose of William Blake,* edited by David V. Erdman with commentary by Harold Bloom. Published by Doubleday and Company, Inc., Garden City, 1970.)

62: Opler. "Childhood and Youth in Jicarilla Apache Society." (See number 45.)

63: Nelson, Edward Wilson. "The Eskimo About Bering Strait." In *Annual Report of the Bureau of American Ethnology: 1896–1897.* Washington, D.C.: Government Printing Office, 1901.

64: Thompson, Robert Farris. *Black Gods and Kings: Yoruba Art at U.C.L.A.* Los Angeles: University of California Museum and Laboratories of Ethnic Arts and Technology, 1971.

65: Hole, Christina. *English Folklore.* London: B. T. Batsford, Ltd., 1940.

66: Bergen. *Current Superstitions from the Oral Tradition of English Speaking Folk.* (See number 37.)

Fogel. *Beliefs and Superstitions of the Pennsylvania Germans.* (See number 37.)

Demetrio, Francisco R. *Dictionary of Philippine Folk Beliefs and Customs.* Cagayan de Oro City: Xavier University, 1970.

67: Trevelyan, Marie. *Folk-Lore and Folk-Stories of Wales.* London: E. Stock, 1909.

68: Gaster. *The Holy and the Profane.* (See number 35.)

69: Elwin. *Folk Songs of Chattisgarh.* (See number 21.)

70: Cirlot, Juan Eduardo. *A Dictionary of Symbols* (translated from Spanish by Jack Sage). NY: Philosophical Library, Inc., 1962.

71: Cavendish, Richard. *The Black Arts.* NY: G. P. Putnam's Sons, 1967.

72: Day, Clarence B. *Chinese Peasant Cults: Being a Study of Chinese Paper Gods.* Shanghai: Kelly and Walsh, Ltd., 1940.

73: Waley, Arthur. *Translations from the Chinese.* NY: Alfred A. Knopf, Inc., 1919.

74: Bunzel, Ruth L. "Zuñi Ritual Poetry." In *The 47th Annual Report of the Bureau of American Ethnology.* Washington, D.C.: Government Printing Office, 1932.

75: Driberg, Jack H. *Initiation: Translations from the Poems of the Didinga and Lango Tribes.* Waltham Saint Lawrence, Berkshires: Golden Cockerel Press, 1932.

76: Leach, Maria, ed. *Funk and Wagnalls Standard Dictionary of Mythology and Folklore.* NY: Funk and Wagnalls Company, 1949. Volume I.

77: Dickens, Charles. *David Copperfield.*

78: Boas, Franz. *The Religion of the Kwakiutl Indians,* Volume II. NY: Columbia University Press, 1930. Published as "Columbia University Contributions to Anthropology," Volume 10.

79: Rexroth, Kenneth, translator. *One Hundred Poems from the Chinese.* NY: New Directions, 1965.

80: Vallat-Emrich, Marion and Korson, George, editors. *The Child's Book of Folklore.* NY: Dial Press, 1947.

81: Rasmussen, Knut. *Intellectual Culture of the Iglulik Eskimos* (Report of the Fifth Thule Expedition 1921–24, Volume VII, Number 1). (Translated by W. Worster.) Copenhagen: Gyldendalske Boghandel, Nordisk Forlag, 1929.

82: Folklore collected by the editor.

83: Mason, Redfern. *The Song Lore of Ireland.* NY: Wessels and Bissell Company, 1910.

84: Seligmann, C. G. and Brenda Z. *The Veddas.* Cambridge: The University Press, 1911.

85: Chamberlin. *The Child and Childhood in Folk-Thought.* (See number 10.)

86: Hahn, Theophilus. "Die Nama-Hottentotten." In *Globus XII.* (1867).

Checklist

NOTE: *The checklist is in two parts. The first list stresses titles which help to further define the feminine aspect in history and culture. The second is a small list of books on child-birthing, but is a basic collection. The emphasis is primarily on natural childbirth.*　　　　D.M.

THE FEMININE ASPECTS

Arguelles, Miriam and Jose. *The Feminine: Spacious as the Sky.* Boulder: Shambhala Publications, 1977.

Ashe, Geoffrey. *The Virgin.* London: Routledge and Kegan Paul,, 1976.

Bachofen, J. J. *Myth, Religion, and Mother Right* (translated by Ralph Manheim). Princeton: Princeton University Press (Bollingen Series LXXXIV), 1967.

Bataille, Georges. *Death and Sensuality: A Study of Eroticism and the Taboo* (translated by Mary Dalwood). NY: Walker and Company, 1962.

Beard, Mary R. *Woman as Force in History: A Study of Traditions and Realities.* NY: Collier, 1971.

de Beauvoir, Simone. *The Second Sex.* NY: Alfred A. Knopf, 1953.

Bell, Susan G., ed. *Women: From the Greeks to the French Revolution.* Belmont: Wadsworth Publishing Company, 1972.

Borgese, Elisabeth Mann. *Ascent of Woman.* NY: George Braziller, 1963.

Bramly, Serge. *Macumba: The Teachings of Maria-José, Mother of the Gods.* NY: St. Martin's Press, 1977.

Brandon, S. G. F. *Creation Legends of the Ancient Near East.* NY: Verry, Lawrence, 1963.

Briffault, Robert. *The Mothers: A Study of the Origins of Sentiments and Institutions.* London and New York: The Macmillan Company, 1927. Three volumes.

Briggs, Katherine M. *The Fairies in the English Tradition.* Chicago: University of Chicago Press, 1967.

Campbell, Joseph. *Hero With a Thousand Faces.* Princeton: Princeton University Press (Bollingen Series XVII), 1968.

———. *The Mythic Image.* Princeton: Princeton University Press (Bollingen Series C), 1975.

Cisneros, Florence Garcia and Rafael Llerena. *Maternity in Pre-Columbian Art.* NY: Cisneros Gallery of New York, 1970.

Clark, Sir Kenneth. *The Nude.* Garden City: Anchor Books, 1959.

Clark, R. T. *Myth and Symbol in Ancient Egypt.* NY: Grove Press, 1960.

Cles-Reden, Sibylle von. *The Realm of the Great Goddess: The Story of the Megalith Builders.* London: Thames and Hudson, 1961.

Crawford, O. G. S. *The Eye Goddess.* London: Phoenix House Limited, 1957.

Dames, Michael. *The Silbury Treasure: The Great Goddess Rediscovered.* London: Thames and Hudson, 1977.

Davies, R. Trevor. *Four Centuries of Witch Belief.* London: Methuen, 1947.

Dawson, W. R. *The Customs of Couvade.* Manchester: Manchester University Press, 1929.

Deren, Maya. *The Divine Horseman.* NY: Chelsea House, 2nd edition, 1970.

Diner, Helen. *Mothers and Amazons: The First Feminine History of Culture* (edited and translated by John Philip Lundlin). NY: The Julian Press, Inc., 1965.

Dinnerstein, Dorothy. *The Mermaid and the Minotaur: Sexual Arrangements and Human Malaise.* NY: Harper and Row, 1976.

D(oolittle), H(ilda). *Helen in Egypt.* NY: Grove Press, 1961.

———. *Hermetic Definition.* NY: New Directions, 1972.

———. *Trilogy.* NY: New Directions, 1973.

———. *Tribute to Freud.* Boston: David R. Godine, 1974.

Drachler, Rose. *The Choice.* Berkeley: Tree Books, 1977.

Drinker, Sophie L. *Music and Women.* NY: Coward-McCann, Inc., 1948.

Ehrenreich, Barbara and Deirdre English. *Witches, Midwives, and Nurses: A History of Women Healers.* NY: The Feminist Press, 1972.

Ellis, Davidson H. R. *Gods and Myths of Northern Europe.* Baltimore: Penguin Books, 1964.

Elworthy, Frederick Thomas. *The Evil Eye.* NY: The Julian Press, Inc., 1958.

Engelmann, Dr. George. *Labor Among Primitive Peoples.* St. Louis: J. H. Chambers and Co., 1883.

Evans-Pritchard, E. E. *The Position of Women in Primitive Societies.* NY: Free Press, 1965.

Findley, Dr. Palmer. *The Story of Childbirth.* Garden City: Doubleday, Doran and Company, Inc., 1933.

Frankfort, Henri. *Ancient Egyptian Religion: An Interpretation.* NY: Harper and Row, 1961.

Frazer, Sir James George. *The Golden Bough: A Study in Magic and Religion.* NY: The Macmillan Co., 1922.

Frisbee, Charlotte Johnson. *Kinaaldá: A Study of the Navaho Girl's Puberty Ceremony.* Middletown: Wesleyan University Press, 1967.

Frobenius, Leo. *The Childhood of Man* (translated by A. H. Keane). Philadelphia: 1909.

Gaster, Theodor H., editor. *The New Golden Bough* by Sir James George Frazer. NY: Criterion Books, 1959.

————. *The Holy and the Profane: Evolution of Jewish Folkways*. NY: William Sloane Associates, Publishers, 1955.

Gifford, Edward S. *The Evil Eye: Studies in the Folklore of Vision*. NY: The Macmillan Co., 1958.

Gimbutas, Marija. *The Gods and Goddesses of Old Europe: 7000 to 3500 B.C., Myths, Legends and Cult Images*. Berkeley: University of California Press, 1974.

Graves, Robert. *The White Goddess*. London: Faber and Faber Ltd., 1948.

Grinnell, Robert. *Alchemy in a Modern Woman: A Study of the Contrasexual Archetype*. NY: Spring Publications, 1973.

Harding, M. Esther. *Women's Mysteries*. NY: G. P. Putnam's Sons, 1971.

Harrison, Jane Ellen. *Prolegomena to the Study of Greek Religion*. NY: Meridian Books, 1955.

————. *Epilegomena to the Study of Greek Religion and Themis: A Study of the Social Origins of Greek Religion*. New Hyde Park: University Books, 1962.

————. *Ancient Art and Ritual*. London: Thornton Butterworth Ltd., 1913.

Hays, H. R. *The Dangerous Sex: The Myth of Feminine Evil*. NY: Simon and Schuster, 1965.

Herschberger, Ruth. *Adam's Rib*. NY: Pellegrini and Cudahy, 1948.

Horner, I. B. *Women Under Primitive Buddhism: Laywomen and Almswomen*. London: George Routledge and Sons, 1930.

Hurston, Zora Neale. *Tell My Horse*. Philadelphia and New York: J. B. Lippincott Company, 1938.

James, E. O. *The Cult of the Mother Goddess: An Archeological and Documentary Study*. NY: Frederick A. Praeger, 1959.

Jonas, Hans. *Gnostic Religion*. Boston: Beacon Press, 1963.

Kerenyi, Carl. *Dionysos: Archetypal Image of Indestructible Life*. Princeton: Princeton University Press (Bollingen Series LXV:2), 1976.

————. *Eleusis: Archetypal Image of Mother and Daughter*. Princeton: Princeton University Press (Bollingen Series LXV:4), 1976.

————. *Zeus and Hera: Archetypal Image of Father, Husband, and Wife*. Princeton: Princeton University Press (Bollingen Series LXV:5), 1975.

Kinsey, Alfred C., Wardell B. Pomeroy, Clyde E. Martin, and Paul H. Gebhard. *Sexual Behavior in the Human Female*. Philadelphia: W. B. Saunders Company, 1953.

Kramer, Samuel Noah. *Sumerian Mythology*. NY: Harper and Row, 1961.

Kyger, Joanne. *All This Every Day*. Bolinas: Big Sky, 1975.

Laing, R. D. and A. Esterson. *Sanity, Madness and the Family*. London: Pelican Books, 1970.

LeSueur, Meridel. *Rites of Ancient Ripening*. Minneapolis: Vanilla Press, 1975.

Levy, Rachel G. *The Gate of Horn*. London: Methuen, 1948.

Lewinsohn, Richard. *A History of Sexual Customs*. NY: Harper and Row, 1971.

Markale, Jean. *Women of the Celts* (translated by A. Mygind, C. Hauch, and P. Henry). London: Gordon-Cremones, 1975.

Mason, Otis T. *Woman's Share in Primitive Culture*. NY: D. Appleton and

Company, 1894.

Murray, Margaret A. *The God of the Witches.* Garden City: Doubleday and Company, 1960.

———. *The Witch-Cult in Western Europe.* Oxford: Oxford University Press, 1967.

Neumann, Erich. *The Great Mother: An Analysis of the Archetype* (translated by Ralph Manheim). Princeton: Princeton University Press (Bollingen Series XLVII), 1970.

———. *Amor and Psyche: The Psychic Development of the Feminine* (translated by Ralph Manheim). Princeton: Princeton University Press (Bollingen Series LIV), 1971.

Newall, Venetia, editor. *The Witch Figure: Essays in Honor of Katherine M. Briggs.* London and Boston: Routledge and Kegan Paul, 1973.

Pagels, Elaine H. *The Gnostic Gospels.* NY: Random House, 1979.

Patai, Raphael. *The Hebrew Goddess.* NY: KTAV Publishing House, 1967.

Pinkham, Mildred Worth. *Women in the Sacred Scriptures of Hinduism.* NY: AMS Press, 1967.

Pomeroy, Sarah B. *Goddesses, Whores, Wives and Slaves: Women in Classical Antiquity.* NY: Schocken Books, 1975.

Power, Eileen. *Medieval Women* (edited by M. Poston). Cambridge: Cambridge University Press, 1976.

Reich, Wilhelm. *The Function of the Orgasm* (translated by Thoedore P. Wolfe). NY: Noonday Press, 1961.

———. *The Sexual Revolution.* NY: Noonday Press, 1963.

Rosaldo, Michelle Zimbalist and Louise Lamphere, editors. *Women, Culture, and Society.* Stanford: Stanford University Press, 1974.

Ross, Anne. *Pagan Celtic Britain: Studies in Iconography and Tradition.* London: Routledge and Kegan Paul; NY: Columbia University Press, 1967.

Rush, Anne Kent. *Moon, Moon.* Berkeley: Moon Books; NY: Random House, 1977.

Schafer, Edward H. *The Divine Woman: Dragon Ladies and Rain Maidens in T'ang Literature.* Berkeley: North Point Press, 1980.

Scheinfeld, Amram. *Twins and Super-Twins.* NY: J. B. Lippincott, 1967.

Solanas, Valerie. *S. C. U. M. Manifesto.* NY: Olympia Press, 1968.

Spence, Lewis. *Gods of Mexico.* London: T. F. Unwin, Limited, 1923.

Stead, Christina. *The Man Who Loved Children.* NY: Holt, Rinehart and Winston, 1965.

Stone, Merlin. *When God Was a Woman.* NY: The Dial Press, 1976.

Turner, Kay, editor. *Lady-Unique-Inclination-of-the-Night* (Cycles 1 through 4). New Brunswick: Lady Unique Collective, 1976–1978.

Von Franz, Maria Louise. *Problems of the Feminine in Fairytales.* NY: Spring Publications, 1972.

———. *Patterns of Creativity Mirrored in Creation Myths.* NY: Spring Publications, 1972.

———. *A Psychological Interpretation of the Golden Ass of Apuleius.* NY: Spring Publications, 1970.

Arms, Suzanne. *Immaculate Deception: A New Look at Women and Childbirth in America*. Boston: Houghton Mifflin, 1975.

Bing, Elisabeth. *Six Practical Lessons for an Easier Childbirth*. NY: Bantam Books, 1969.

Boston Women's Collective. *Our Bodies Ourselves*. NY: Simon and Schuster, 1972.

Davis, Adelle. *Let's Have Healthy Children*. NY: Harcourt, Brace and World, 1972. Second Edition Revised.

Dick-Read, Grantly, M.D. *Childbirth Without Fear: The Principles and Practice of Natural Childbirth*. NY: Harper and Row, 1970.

Eloesser, Leo, Edith J. Galt and Isabel Hemingway. *Pregnancy, Childbirth and the Newborn: A Manual for Rural Midwives*. Mexico City: Instituto Indigenista Interamericano, 1959.

Gaskin, Ina May. *Spiritual Midwifery*. Summertown: The Book Publishing Company, 1978.

Guttmacher, Alan F., M.D. *Pregnancy and Birth: A Book for Expectant Parents*. NY: Signet Books, 1962.

Hazell, Lester Dessez. *Commonsense Childbirth*. NY: Berkeley Medallion Books, 1976.

Kippley, Sheila. *Breast-Feeding and Natural Child Spacing: The Ecology of Natural Mothering*. NY: Harper and Row, 1974.

Lamaze, Dr. Fernand. *Painless Childbirth: The Lamaze Method*. NY: Pocket Books, 1972.

Leboyer, Frederick. *Birth Without Violence*. NY: Alfred A. Knopf, 1975.

Miller, John Seldon, M.D. *Childbirth: A Manual for Pregnancy and Delivery*. NY: Atheneum, 1971.

Nilsson, Lennart. *A Child Is Born: The Drama of Life Before Birth*. NY: Delacorte Press, 1966.

Sousa, Marion. *Childbirth at Home*. NY: Bantam Books, 1977.

(continued from copyright page)

Aboriginal Myths and Legends, by Roland Robinson. Reprinted with permission of Macmillan Company of Australia Pty Ltd. *The Legends of the Jews*, Volume I and II, by Louis Ginzberg. This material is copyrighted by and used through the courtesy of the Jewish Publication Society of America. *Man: Grand Symbol of the Mysteries*, by Manly P. Hall. Published by The Philosophical Research Society, Inc. Reprinted by permission. *Buddhist Scriptures*, translated and edited by Edward Conze. Copyright © 1959 Edward Conze. Reprinted by permission of Penguin Books Ltd. "Egyptian Rituals and Incantations," and "Egyptian Hymns and Prayers," both translated by John A. Wilson, and "Akkadian Myths and Epics," translated by John A. Speiser in *Ancient Near Eastern Texts Relating to the Old Testament* by James B. Pritchard (ed.), 3rd ed. with Supplement (Copyright © 1969 by Princeton University Press), pp. 328, 370, and 100, part of which is in paraphrased form. Reprinted by permission of Princeton University Press. *Tarzan Alive*, by Philip José Farmer. Copyright © 1972 Philip José Farmer. Reprinted by permission of Doubleday and Company, Inc. *The Life of Apollonius of Tyana*, Philostratus. Translated by F. C. Conybeare. Published by Harvard University Press. Reprinted by permission of Harvard University Press. *Ancilla to Pre-Socratic Philosophers*, translated and edited by Kathleen Freeman. Published by Harvard University Press. Reprinted by permission. *The Midwife and the Witch*, by Thomas Roger Forbes. Copyright © 1966 Thomas Roger Forbes. Published by Yale University Press. Reprinted by permission. *The Tibetan Book of the Dead or the After-Death Experiences on the Bardo Plane* by W. Y. Evans-Wentz. Copyright © 1960 by W. Y. Evans-Wentz. Reprinted by permission of Oxford University Press, Inc. "The Stork and Babies," in *How Did It Begin?*, by Rudolph Brasch. Published by David McKay Co. Reprinted by permission of the author. *Conversations with Ogotemmêli: An Introduction to Dogon Religious Ideas*, by Marcel Griaule. (Translated by Daryll Forde.) Published by Oxford University Press for The International African Institute, 1965. *The Search for the Beloved*, by Nandor Fodor (1949); *Amulets and Talismans*, by E. A. Wallis Budge (1961); *The 100 Thousand Songs of Milarepa*, by Garma C. C. Chang. All reprinted by permission of University Books, Inc. Published by arrangement with Lyle Stuart. *Folk Songs of Chattisgarh*, translated and edited by Verrier Elwin. Reprinted by permission of Oxford University Press. *Life in a Haitian Valley*, by Melville J. Herskovits. Copyright © 1937 by Alfred A. Knopf, Inc. and renewed 1965 by Frances S. Herskovits. Reprinted by permission of Alfred A. Knopf, Inc. "On the Birth of His Son," in *Translations from the Chinese*, translated by Arthur Waley. Copyright © 1919 and renewed 1947 by Arthur Waley. Reprinted by permission of Alfred A. Knopf, Inc. *Santeria: African Magic in Latin America*, by Migene Gonzalez-Wippler. Published by Julian Press, Inc., A Division of Crown Publishers, Inc., 1973. Reprinted by permission of the author. *The Evil Eye*, by Edward S. Gifford, Jr. Copyright © Edward S. Gifford, Jr. 1956, 1957, 1958. Reprinted with permission of Macmillan Publishing Co., Inc. "Adam and Eve: Lilith, avaunt! Sinoi, Sinsinol, and S-m-n-g-l-f" and "The Tree of Life" from *The Holy and the Profane*, Rev. Ed., by Theodor H. Gaster. Copyright © 1955, 1980 by Theodor H. Gaster. Reprinted by permission of William Morrow & Company. *Ozark Superstitions*, by Vance Randolph. Reprinted by permission of Columbia University Press. "Popular Beliefs & Practices from Alabama," in *Folklore Studies: 9* (1958), Ray B. Browne. Reprinted by permission of The University of California Press. "Folklore of Pregnancy: Wives' Tales in Contra Costa County, California," by Lucile F. Newman, in *Western Folklore*, Vol. 28, #23, 1969. Reprinted by permission of the California Folklore Society. *Folk-Lore from Adams County, Illinois*, by Harry Middleton Hyatt. The Alma Egan Hyatt Foundation, 1935. *Sanskrit Poetry from Vidyakara's "Treasury,"* translated and edited by Daniel H. H. Ingalls. Copyright © 1965, 1968 by The President and Fellows of Harvard College. Published by Harvard University Press. Reprinted by permission. *The Great Mother: An Analysis of the Archetype,* translated by Ralph Manheim, Bollingen Series XLVII. Copyright © 1955 by Princeton University Press. Published by Princeton University Press. Reprinted by permission of Princeton University Press. "The Couvade," in *Mothers and Amazons: The First Feminine History of Culture,* by Helen Diner. Copyright © 1965 by Julian Press, Inc. Used by permission of Julian Press, Inc., A Division of Crown Publishers, Inc. *The Old-Fashioned Woman: Primitive Fancies About the Sex,* by Elsie Clews Parsons. Copyright © 1913 G. P. Putnam's Sons. Published by G. P. Putnam's Sons. Reprinted by permission. "Childhood and Youth in Jicarilla Apache Society," by Morris E. Opler, in *Publications of the Frederick Webb Hodge Society Publication Fund,* Volume 5 (1946). Reprinted by permission of the Southwest Museum. *Maternity and Its Rituals in Bang Chan,* by Jane Richardson Hanks, in Cornell University Southeast Asia Program Data Paper #51, Cornell Thailand Project Interim Reports Series Number Six, 1963. Reprinted by permission of The Cornell University Southeast Asia Program. *The Story of the Nursery,* by Magdalen King-Hall. Published by Routledge & Kegan Paul. Reprinted by permission of the Estate of Magdalen King-Hall. "Hawaiian Beliefs and Customs During Birth, Infancy and Childhood," by Mary Kawena Pukui, in *Occasional Papers of the Bernice P. Bishop Museum,* Volume 16, Number 17, March 20, 1942. Reprinted by permission of The Bishop Museum Press. *Life Begins: Childbirth in Lore and its Literature,* by Morris Braude. Argus Books, Chicago, 1935. *Songs and Tales of the Sea Kings,* by Frank J. Stimson. Published by The Peabody Museum of Salem. Reprinted through the courtesy of The Peabody Museum of Salem, Massachusetts. *Baba of Karo: A Woman of the Moslem Hausa,* by Mary Smith. Published by Frederick A. Praeger. 1964. Copyright 1954 by Faber and Faber LTD. Reprinted by permission of Faber and Faber LTD. "My Mother's Womb," by Blaise Cendrars. Translated from the French by Denis Kelly. "How an Unborn Child Avenged its Mother's Death," in *African Folktales and Sculpture,* ed. Paul Radin and James Johnson Sweeney, Bollingen Series XXXII. Copyright © 1954, 1964 by Princeton University Press. Reprinted by permission of Princeton University Press. "Some Observations & Customs of the Mansi (Voguls) in Connection with Childbirth," by E. I. Rombandeeva, in *Popular Beliefs and Folklore Traditions in Siberia,* edited V. Dioszegi. Published and reprinted by permission of The Uralic and Altaic Series, Indiana University, Bloomington and The Hungarian Academy of Sciences, Budapest. *Black Gods and Kings: Yoruba Art at U.C.L.A.,* by Robert Farris Thompson. University of California Museum and Laboratories of Ethnic Arts and Technology, 1971. Reprinted by permission of Robert Farris Thompson, Yale University. *English Folklore,* by Christina Hole. Published by Batsford Limited. (1940). Reprinted by permission of B. T. Batsford Ltd. *Dictionary of Philippine Folk Beliefs and Customs,* by Francisco R. Demetrio. Published by Xavier University, Cagayan de Oro City, R. P., Volume IV, #2253. Reprinted by permission of Xavier University. *A Dictionary of Symbols,* by Juan Cirlot, translated from the Spanish by Jack Sage. Published by Philosophical Library. Reprinted by permission. *The Black Arts,* by Richard Cavendish. Copyright © 1967 by Richard Cavendish. Reprinted by permission of G. P. Putnam's Sons. *Initiation: Translations from the Poems of the Didinga and Lango Tribes,* by Jack H. Driberg. Published by Golden Cockerel Press. Reprinted by permission. "Caul," in *Standard Dictionary of Folklore, Mythology and Legend,* edited by Maria Leach (Funk & Wagnalls). Copyright © 1972, 1950, 1949, by Harper & Row Publishers, Inc. Reprinted by permission of the Publisher. *The Religion of the Kwakiutl Indians,* by Franz Boas. "Columbia University Contributions to Anthropology," Volume 10. Columbia University

Press, 1930. Reprinted by permission of Columbia University Press. *One Hundred Poems from the Chinese*, translated by Kenneth Rexroth. All Rights Reserved. Copyright © 1971 by Kenneth Rexroth. Reprinted by permission of New Directions. *The Child's Book of Folklore*, edited by Marion Vallat-Emrich and George Korson. Published by Dial Press, 1947. Reprinted by permission of Mrs. George Korson. *The Veddas*, by C. G. and Brenda Z. Seligmann. Published by Cambridge University Press. Reprinted by permission of Cambridge University Press. *Intellectual Culture of the Iglulik Eskimos* (Report of the Fifth Thule Expedition 1921–1924, Volume VII, Number 1), by Knut Rasmussen, translated by W. Worster. Published by Gyldendalske Boghandel, Nordisk Forlag.

Design by David Bullen
Typeset in 10pt Caledonia
by Accent & Alphabet
Printed by Maple-Vail
on acid-free paper